Medicare Matters

CALIFORNIA/MILBANK BOOKS ON HEALTH AND THE PUBLIC

Medicare Matters

What Geriatric Medicine Can Teach
American Health Care

Christine K. Cassel

University of California Press
BERKELEY / LOS ANGELES / LONDON

Milbank Memorial Fund
NEW YORK

The Milbank Memorial Fund is an endowed operating foundation that engages in nonpartisan analysis, study, research, and communication on significant issues in health policy. In the Fund's own publications, in reports or books it publishes with other organizations, and in articles it commissions for publication by other organizations, the Fund endeavors to maintain the highest standards for accuracy and fairness. Statements by individual authors, however, do not necessarily reflect opinions or factual determinations of the Fund.

University of California Press
Berkeley and Los Angeles, California

University of California Press, Ltd.
London, England

Library of Congress Cataloging-in-Publication Data

Cassel, Christine K.
    Medicare matters : what geriatric medicine can teach American health care / Christine K. Cassel.
        p.   ;   cm. — (California/Milbank books on health and the public ; 14)
    Includes bibliographical references and index.
    ISBN 0-520-24624-1 (cloth : alk. paper)
    1. Medicare.   2. Geriatrics—United States.   3. Medical policy—United States.   4. Older people—Medical care—United States.
    [DNLM: 1. Medicare   2. Geriatrics—United States.   3. Health policy—United States.   4. Health Services for the Aged—United States.
    WT 31 C344m 2005]   I. Cassel, Christine K.   II. Series.
        RA412.3.C39 2005
        368.4'26'00973—dc22   2005011748

Manufactured in the United States of America
14   13   12   11   10   09   08   07   06   05
10   9   8   7   6   5   4   3   2   1

This book is printed on New Leaf EcoBook 60, containing 60% post-consumer waste, processed chlorine free; 30% de-inked recycled fiber, elemental chlorine free; and 10% FSC-certified virgin fiber, totally chlorine free. EcoBook 60 is acid-free and meets the minimum requirements of ANSI/ASTM D5634–01 (*Permanence of Paper*).

To Bernice Neugarten,
founder of the field of social gerontology,
and to Paul Beeson, who lit the spark
that created geriatric medicine
in the United States

Contents

Foreword

The Milbank Memorial Fund is an endowed operating foundation that engages in nonpartisan analysis, study, research, and communication on significant issues in health policy. Since 1905 the Fund has worked to improve and maintain health by encouraging persons who make and implement health policy to use the best available evidence. The Fund convenes meetings of leaders in the public and private sectors and publishes reports, articles, and books.

This is the fourteenth of the California/Milbank Books on Health and the Public. The publishing partnership between the Fund and the University of California Press seeks to encourage the synthesis and communication of findings from research that could contribute to more effective health policy.

In *Medicare Matters* Christine K. Cassel discusses policy for organizing and financing Medicare in the context of the best available evidence about preventing and treating the illnesses of elderly persons and managing their care. Cassel describes how policy for Medicare has affected the health of beneficiaries in the past and recommends changes in policy that could contribute to improving their health in the future.

Cassel believes that policy for Medicare must be informed by franker and more thorough public discussion about what she calls the "social contract on which our government is based." American society, she persuasively argues, should be a "good place for all generations." Achieving this goal requires better public understanding of the complementary responsibilities of government and the private sector.

The book is informed by Cassel's experience as a clinician, educator, researcher, leader in internal medicine and the subspecialty of geriatric medicine, and frequent adviser to policy makers. She makes that experience accessible in this book, augmenting it by broad as well as deep reading in the literature of clinical medicine and health policy.

Daniel M. Fox
President

Samuel L. Milbank
Chairman

Preface

This book has undergone a very extended gestation. It began in discussions with Dan Fox, president of the Milbank Memorial Fund, more than five years ago, as we shared observations about how Medicare fails to create incentives for—or even the possibility of—the changes in health care made necessary by both advanced medical science and an aging population. To me, a physician caring for elderly patients and an educator teaching medical students and residents in geriatric medicine, the misfit between what I was teaching as an ideal model for care of the elderly and what my students and residents were finding when they began to practice became more glaring with each passing year.

With these observations, the germ of this book took hold.

At the same time there was a growing awareness, outlined trenchantly by Jonathan Oberlander in *The Political Life of Medicare,* that the societal and political consensus supporting a universal health insurance risk pool and public financial support for medical care for the elderly was beginning to unravel. Herein there is a paradox. As an insurance plan, Medicare does not create the environment needed for the practice of high-quality modern geriatric medicine. On the other hand, Medicare is much better health insurance than a large majority of Americans now enjoy. Indeed, during many of the recent health-care reform movements, I have often heard younger people exclaim, "If we could just have Medicare!"

In the simplicity of its administration and the universality of its risk pool, Medicare is a model for universal health insurance. Yet it is also in desperate need of modernization: Congress must initiate any change to benefits outside of demonstration plans or waivers, placing Medicare in a fee-for-service straitjacket. Considering the complexity of political debates, the ideological charge of disputes about the appropriate role of government in the private lives of American citizens, and the rapid growth of the health-care industry, it is no wonder that the average citizen is confused about whether and to what degree Medicare really matters.

I wrote this book because I believe that Medicare does matter—not just to the elderly and not just to the health-care providers who care for them, but to our entire society. It matters because it is the only model we have of universal health insurance, and it matters because Medicare provides benefits not only to the elderly, but also to families in which older people depend on children, grandchildren, and great-grandchildren for support. This is particularly true as life expectancy increases and as women outlive the support of their husbands and pensions. Older people can benefit and contribute to society if they have access to effective medical care. The same medical care, if fostered by good insurance, can free adult children to support their own children rather than worrying about how they will pay for the care of elderly parents. Thus, I hope this book will find its way into the hands of thoughtful people from all walks of life and of all ages. I hope especially to speak to the baby boom generation, of which I am a member. We aren't yet eligible for Medicare, but it is in our interest to be looking ahead at what Medicare can provide us as we get older and what it means to our children and grandchildren—and indeed, what it means to our communities and our nation.

During the time this book was written, we have witnessed drastic changes in our political environment and intense debates about the future of Medicare. But the fundamental points in this book are not altered by the Medicare Modernization Act or by other changes at the edges of Medicare. Some of the examples I use to illustrate points will inevitably be dated as new legislation is enacted, but the reality remains consistent: Medicare regulation is too complex, the benefit package is too inconsistent, and most payment models are too inflexible to foster effective geriatric care.

In addition to the thanks I offer Dan Fox for his ongoing support, unwavering critical attention, and innovative thinking, I owe a debt of gratitude to research assistants Lydia Siegel, Beth Demel, Terry Hammond, and Linda Rosen. I also owe gratitude to a number of people who gave me wonderful critical advice, including Marilyn Moon, Edward Lawlor, Carroll Estes, Joanne Lynn, Murray Ross, John Rother, Ruth Purtilo, Robert Berenson, Judith Hibbard, Arthur Levin, Corrine Rieder, Robyn Stone, and Lynne Withey—thoughtful, smart, experienced people who have different views on specific aspects of Medicare policy, but who agree with me about its fundamental importance to making a success of our aging society.

Introduction

Many books about Medicare are published every year. Medicare's size, its cost, and its centrality to the American health-care system have made it a subject of consistent interest to policy analysts, political pundits, and the public. The Medicare Prescription Drug Improvement and Modernization Act of 2003 (MMA) is spawning even more new publications about Medicare. This book is different: I write as a physician who has spent an entire career caring for elderly Medicare patients. My career has spanned almost the entire duration of modern Medicare, and I have witnessed the affection and disdain, concern and celebration, and attack and protection directed toward the Medicare program over more than thirty years. I have written this book because I believe that modern geriatric medicine holds the secret of how to sustain and improve health care for older people in our society. Even more powerfully, geriatric medicine, and its application to the Medicare population, provides important lessons for dealing with the chronic problems of the American health-care system and thus providing all Americans, no matter what age, with high-quality and affordable health care.

Medicare matters because it is the key to a health-care policy that can serve not only the increasing proportion of older people in the United States but entire families. Medicare matters because it can help us balance the roles of the public and private sectors in the centrally important issue of health care. And it matters because it represents one aspect of the fundamental social contract on which our nation is built. By understanding Medicare, we can see with clarity what a commitment to good government can accomplish and how collective approaches to big social problems can create a society in which all can thrive.

A key feature of the 2003 Medicare legislation is its emphasis on private plans, both in implementing the drug benefit and in providing an incentive to managed-care plans to participate more fully in the Medicare program. The new drug benefit provides little real help to elders either in getting better value for money or in covering the cost of their medications. But it is important because it illustrates the highly political nature of Medicare policy making and the unreliable cost projections that are the basis for policy decisions. If we understand the inevitably political nature of debates on Medicare, we can challenge our political system to deal honestly and effectively with real problems and to devise solutions based on accurate information about costs and the effectiveness of medical treatments.

This legislation fails to address all of the problems with the current Medicare system or the critical challenge of defining and providing effective health care for an aging population in the American political landscape. These are the issues that my patients and I live and breathe every day. I firmly believe that we can find answers to the problems of Medicare if we look beyond political rhetoric.

What Matters?

The aging of the baby boomers is now old news. In all of the media chatter devoted to it, however, are some fundamental and remarkable truths. The dramatic advances in longevity that have occurred over just the last century are unprecedented in the history of the human species. Between 1900 and 2000, life expectancy at birth in the United States increased from 47 to 77 years, a change mirrored in most of the developed world. Life expectancy for people aged 65 increased more than 6 years during the twentieth century; in 2002, a 65-year-old American woman could expect to live almost 20 more years, and a man an additional 16.6 years. These changes readily illustrate why the issue of population aging is so complex and why the problem of providing medical care for an aging population cannot be addressed with one or two simple policy steps.

It is important to keep in mind that increased longevity is very good news. We hear so much about the burdens of Medicare expenditures and Social Security costs that we may forget our remarkable good fortune at living in the twenty-first century, when most of us can expect to live to an advanced old age and to remain reasonably healthy and functional. This is a miracle attributable to the combination of modern civilization and our growing understanding of what keeps people healthy. Some of our increasing longevity, but not by any stretch most or all of it, is due to medical care.

Population aging affects entire families. The elderly, whether seen as the deserving beneficiaries of government programs or as "greedy geezers" soaking up resources that could be used for younger people, are members of families. Instead of the traditional three generations of grandparents, parents, and children, today's families may include four and even five generations. Older people contribute personal care and affection, as well as financial resources, to the fabric of families. If the needs of these multigenerational families are not met by a collective social contract, adult children must shoulder the considerable burden of supporting the elders in the family when frailty strikes. That is how families work. (Older people tend to see themselves not as members of a "generation" but rather as part of a "family.") Expenditures on caring for a disabled person, whether an older person or a child, consume resources that the family might otherwise use to better their children's education and to maintain their quality of life.

We have much to learn from looking at the experiences of other countries that began to confront the "crisis" of caring for an aging population ten or even twenty years ago. The United States is by no means the world leader in longevity. For life expectancy at birth, it is ranked twenty-fourth among males and twenty-first among females, behind Japan and most Western European countries. In terms of life expectancy at age sixty-five, the United States ranks thirteenth for males and fourteenth for females, once again trailing Japan and Western Europe. While there are clear similarities in health-care services among most European countries, Japan, and the United States, there is also a critical difference: all except the United States provide their citizens with universal health insurance. The richest nation on earth has not been able to do this. We argue that the costs are too great and that we disagree about the appropriate role of government in solving these problems. But, interestingly, the idea of the social contract allows countries with very different political systems and economic situations to support universal access to care. To do so, a government must make a basic commitment to distribute the costs of health risk among the entire population and recognize access to health care as a basic opportunity on which a vigorous private sector relies. In chapter 12, I explore these concepts in more detail, examining political beliefs and slogans that block clear thinking about how to relieve families of the burden of health-care costs and allow all families the advantage of optimal health and the opportunity to participate freely and productively in society.

Discussions of Medicare rely on extensive data, much of it generated by the single-payer system that keeps track of all Medicare services delivered and paid for. Complementary data describes the age, health status, and socioeconomic characteristics of the elderly and disabled who are eligible for Medicare services. The most up-to-date resources for graphic displays of such data are the *2005 Chartbook on Medicare,* available from the Commonwealth Fund, and the publication compiled by Sheila Leatherman and Douglas McCarthy, *Quality of Health Care for Medicare Beneficiaries: A Chartbook.*[1]

The Terms of the Debate

To get beyond Washington-speak and look at what medical care, financed by Medicare, can realistically do to help all of us stay healthier as we grow older, we need to understand the terms of the debate. The two major issues are financing and political philosophy. With regard to financing, the two major concerns of politicians—the costs to consumers and the accelerating costs of health-care commodities—are on a collision course.

FINANCING

The most important group of consumers is made up of Medicare beneficiaries and their families. These consumers pay significant out-of-pocket costs, which will rise further under the new Medicare legislation. When concern about costs reaches a high enough level, political forces are activated and politicians start to pay attention.

A second group of consumers that draws the attention of political leaders is comprised of the businesses that pay for health insurance—for some of their employees, some of the time. Employers have been the traditional funders of health care outside Medicare and have also contributed to the costs of Medigap coverage (insurance for what Medicare doesn't cover) through retirement policies for employees. The United States is the only major industrial country that depends so heavily on employers for health-insurance coverage. But as health-care costs continue to increase, businesses cannot absorb them. This is especially true in the global marketplace, where U.S. businesses are at a disadvantage compared with those in countries where the government funds health care. Employers are increasingly unwilling to pay employee health-insurance premiums when they increase by double-digit percentages each year. They have two choices: to stop offering health-care coverage to their employees—an option that has led to a rise in the number of uninsured people in the United States—or to reduce the amount that they contribute to health insurance. They also are much less willing to provide retiree coverage to fill in the gaps in Medicare. As employers limit their health-care costs in these ways, out-of-pocket expenses increase for patients and their families. Americans report to pollsters that they would be willing to pay higher taxes to reduce the unpredictable burden of out-of-pocket medical expenses, but because political leaders have been focused only on reducing taxes, comprehensive health insurance or even Medicare improvements have been unattainable.

The second aspect of the financing challenge is the degree to which the cost of health care in the United States, including Medicare, is driven by the rapidly rising prices of health-care commodities. While this point may seem obvious, it is sometimes obscured in the debate. Pharmaceutical prices are a good example (though not the only one) of accelerating costs. Patients in the United States pay two to three times as much for most drugs as residents of other countries. The pharmaceutical industry is a powerful force lobbying Congress, makes major contributions to both political parties, and invokes the sacred cow of the "free market" to back up its arguments that no constraints should be placed on drug prices. And yet every other country in the world negotiates with these same drug companies (most of which operate worldwide) for significant reductions in price because they are advocating on behalf of large numbers of their citizens.

In a truly free market, large consumer groups should have more bargaining power. But the 2003 Medicare legislation actually forbids Medicare from bargaining—on behalf of thirty-five million Americans—for drug prices that are comparable to those paid by consumers in other developed countries. The drug industry says that it cannot sustain innovation if we reduce prices; but even throughout the long recession of 2000–2004, many drug companies continued to post double-digit profit margins and rising share prices. Clearly, some compromise must be possible in which profits are reduced somewhat in order to keep prices manageable. Pharmaceutical companies may be able to compensate for price reductions with increased sales as more people have access to needed medications.

Health care is a very profitable business in the United States. With a few important and notable exceptions, we have been unable or unwilling as a society to develop an approach to health care that encourages cost-effective choices and reduces unnecessary, expensive treatments. For example, there are 4.8 times as many coronary angioplasties per capita performed in the United States as in Canada. The United States performs three times as many MRI scans per capita as Canada. Yet such treatments and procedures do not make Americans obviously healthier than our Canadian neighbors. Indeed, Canadians live longer and have better population health measures than Americans do. Americans are opposed to health-care rationing, and any politician who suggests it risks being thrown out of office. And yet health-services research persuasively demonstrates that many of the most expensive treatments in American medical care contribute more to somebody's pocketbook than to a patient's health. There is so much good that modern medicine can do that we must, as a society, accept the need to set limits and examine cost-effectiveness.

PHILOSOPHY

Why does the United States lag behind other countries in longer life expectancy and in providing comprehensive and coordinated systems of care? Why, for example, can't we provide universal entitlement to long-term care at home or in a nursing home?

One answer lies in our political philosophy. The United States was founded on the basis of a social contract, first articulated in the eighteenth century by Enlightenment philosophers, that supports the maximum liberty for each consistent with the maximum liberty for all. This means that each of us is allowed freedoms as long as those freedoms do not impinge on the freedoms of others. And the social contract means that we contribute our resources, by means of local, state, and federal taxes, only to pay for services and protections for the public good, services that government can provide more effectively than the private sector can. Some examples are fire and police services, public highways, sewage treatment, and a basic public-health infrastructure. It would be ridiculous to expect every private citizen to pay only for that piece of road he or she uses to travel to work every day. It is government services like these that allow for a stable civil society.

Health care is most appropriately regarded as belonging in this category of public good. No one knows what their future health-care needs will be, and all citizens are affected equally when these needs are not met. The best way to make sure that adequate resources are available is not to have each person pay out of pocket for their health care but rather to spread the risk across the entire population so that all of us pay a small amount, even though only a relatively small number will actually use those resources. This is the fundamental basis of insurance and of the social contract for all of the public goods just described. Most of us, thankfully, will never need the fire department or police department; but, if we did, we would not want to have to pay them before they agreed to put out a fire, rescue us, or prevent a crime from occurring.

Americans seem to have lost confidence in the ability of government to manage important programs and some are thus reluctant to pay for such programs through taxes. Many appear to believe it is more cost-effective to have health care provided entirely by private entities, and selected and paid for directly by the consumer.

The idea of a marketplace for healthcare, however, is an imperfect idea at best, and to hold Medicare to the standards of a free market is particularly difficult. In health care, a successful free market requires that consumers—whether individual patients or businesses purchasing insurance for their employees—be capable of determining and choosing the lowest cost and the highest quality. Yet our ability to do so is limited by the complexity of health-care issues and the circumstances under which we seek care. How many of us really shop around for the best bargain when we need to have cancer surgery or a Caesarean section? The demands of consumers and of government regulators should indeed lead to better care, and I discuss that issue more in chapter 3. But relying solely on the marketplace forces people who are sick and vulnerable to fend for themselves in a market of very imperfect information. It drives insurance companies to avoid covering people who need health care the most. It means that medical expenses may dramatically affect the ability of a family to support their children's education. These outcomes are not good for the economy and do not lead to effective pressures to contain and reduce health-care costs.

Medicare as a health insurance program has many flaws, mostly attributable to the fact that it is a benefit system designed and administered by Congress rather than by health-care experts. Thus, it falls victim to lobbying groups, special interests, and arbitrary decisions about what is covered and what is not. But Medicare has the lowest administrative costs of any health insurance system in the United States, in many cases by a factor of ten or more. Medicare administrative costs are approximately 3 percent of total Medicare expenditures, whereas private insurance companies often spend between fifteen and thirty cents of each health-care dollar on administrative expenses and profit. So there are some important efficiencies to be gained from a government program. Political slogans about "reducing big government" and "supporting a free market" should not be allowed to obscure the fact that Medicare spends substantially more of each health-care dollar on health services than private insurers do.

Changing the Terms

To reach an informed decision about how best to offer health care to an aging population, we need to change the terms of the debate. It should begin with a discussion of what works, and the answer to this question can be found in the small but important medical specialty of geriatric medicine. Introduced in chapter 1 and discussed more fully in chapter 3, geriatric medicine is based on an understanding of the aging process, the need to prevent disease and disability as we age, and the best ways to care for those who confront the multiple and often chronic disorders related to aging. It is a relatively new specialty in the United States but has had a dramatic effect on our understanding of how best to provide care for older people. Geriatric medicine, as described in chapter 3, is consistent with the ideas promulgated by the Institute of Medicine[2] that have fostered concerns from the public and health care leaders about the gaps in quality of care and patient safety in the United States.

We know that even if we can control costs, health care will be a major expenditure for patients and taxpayers. It is critical to get the best value for our money. The solution to this challenge is the comprehensive approach offered by modern geriatric medicine: well-coordinated care by an interdisciplinary team of health-care professionals. Unfortunately, the Medicare program—because it has been driven by political forces and lobbying groups—does not support such a model. The 2003 Medicare legislation, which pressures consumers to opt for private plans, recognizes that current fee-for-service Medicare fails to provide the care that elderly people really need. Yet the private health-insurance marketplace is not necessarily the best alternative. We need to look very carefully at what constitutes good managed care and consider how to educate American views of this important model.

Good palliative care is an essential feature of modern geriatric medicine. Chapter 5 shows how recent advances in palliative care have enhanced the potential for dignity and relief of suffering at the end of life. Chapter 6 reviews how Medicare decides what treatments and services are paid for and how the political process can create incentives for unnecessary use of expensive technology but not for coordination and communication between different specialists or with patients and families. Here is where good managed care can allow more flexibility. Chapter 7 examines the arbitrariness of starting Medicare coverage at age sixty-five — too early to really be just for frail elderly people and too late to offer preventive care for middle-aged people that could lead to healthier aging.

Chapter 8 examines Medicare financing, which underlies the intensely political nature of the Medicare program since its inception, which in turn is the topic of chapter 10. Prescription drugs, discussed in chapter 9, are essential to modern geriatric medicine and, even with the MMA of 2003, cost more in the United States than in any other country. A better approach to medication coverage is essential for good geriatric care. Of course, the complex world of health policy may be summarized by two questions: who will pay, and how much? The inevitability of some form of rationing of care is described in chapter 11. Finally, chapter 12 returns to the critical importance of the social contract in Medicare matters. An aging society must cater to the needs of all generations.

If Americans can see the benefits of good managed care for the elderly, understand the value of evidence-based models, negotiate for the best prices, set limits on expensive treatments of dubious therapeutic value, and support good geriatric medicine, then the result will be a better approach to health care for *all* Americans. This was Medicare's initial goal in 1965, and it is my deepest hope that in the twenty-first century we might finally achieve it.

CHAPTER I

Medicare and the Social Contract

Medicare is a national social insurance program that provides medical in-surance coverage to about forty million seniors (aged sixty-five and over) and people with disabilities in the United States. The program is seen var-iously as a successful model for universal health coverage and an example of everything that is wrong with a centralized program run by the gov-ernment. Beneficiaries view it as a both godsend and a nightmare.

Medicare has been in existence for almost forty years, long enough to become an established feature of American government: people now ex-pect it to be there for them when they become old or disabled. Many people mistakenly assume that Medicare will cover all of their health-care needs and are surprised and disappointed when they discover the gaps in coverage, particularly for long-term care, chronic care, and medications. Medical professionals may be equally at sea, navigating a system that often fails to meet the contingencies of medical practice and conscientious caregiving. For those trained in geriatric medicine and familiar with the aging process, managing the needs of older people with multiple chronic illnesses and complex care plans within the rules and limits of Medicare can be especially frustrating.

The apparent deficiencies of Medicare look less alarming when com-pared to the poor performance of the rest of the health-care system in the United States, which is reaching a crisis point in terms of both costs and access to care. Medicare, by contrast, has often demonstrated remarkable leadership and ingenuity. The deficiencies we observe in the public pro-gram are related less to government administration than to the immaturity of the private medical and insurance systems on which Medicare is based. The purpose of this book is to accurately characterize Medicare as it exists today, affirm why it matters now more than ever, and suggest some definite ways we might improve it.

A Simple Story

In his recent book *Chaos to Care,* David Lawrence tells the story of the Esther Project in Sweden, which galvanized the medical community there to reorganize and promote coordinated care. Esther, who is eighty-seven years old, lives alone and suffers from congestive heart failure and other ailments. A daughter lives nearby and looks in three times a week. But the kindly old face looking directly at you from Esther's picture is really an actress, a fictional character created by medical leaders to illustrate a common situation: an elderly person with numerous ailments requires coordinated physical, social, and moral support as well as medicine. Esther's story is well known; her picture appears in planning documents and posters; and, according to Lawrence, when "medical professionals and officials talk about redesigning medical care, they refer to Esther."[1]

I present other stories throughout this book. Some are drawn from actual experiences, others are composites drawn from many sources. All of them aim to ground abstract policy discussion in the experiences of individuals like our relatives and friends.

One of my first experiences in geriatric medicine is worth recounting to explain why geriatric medicine differs from what most Americans accept as standard care. In 1980, as a fellow in one of the first geriatric training programs in the United States, I was based at the Veterans Administration (VA) hospital in Portland, Oregon. Many of our patients were World War I veterans, most of them in their eighties. Many were rural men living on farms in eastern Oregon, who rode the bus for three hours to see doctors at the VA. Their medical care was free. They were eligible for Medicare but had been coming to the VA since before Medicare was created and were loyal to the system they knew, though they were often frustrated by fragmented services.

When we started the geriatric clinic, the veterans applauded it. One told me he previously had to spend his entire bus ride into Portland trying to decide which "chief complaint" to express at this visit. The chief complaint is an essential part of how young doctors learn to assess a patient visit: write down the chief complaint in the patient's own words, develop a history of the illness, and then describe the subsequent examination. The problem for most of these elderly veterans was that they had multiple chronic diseases. A single chief complaint did not begin to describe their medical needs. Geriatric medicine recognizes this reality. As one patient said, "Now I can have more than one chief complaint!"

The geriatric clinic also allowed patients to receive a generalist assessment. Most academic hospitals at that time, and many today, are based on specialties; so a patient with a headache might go to a neurology clinic, a patient with joint pain might need to decide whether to go to a rheumatologist or an orthopedist, and a woman with abdominal pain might go to a gastroenterologist even though a gynecologist might be a better choice. Through assessment by a geriatrician, the individual gets appropriate referrals to specialty care and coordinated attention to multiple ailments. The patients at the VA recognized the advantages of the system immediately.

Geriatric Medicine

Geriatric medicine first emerged as a specialty in the early part of the twentieth century. In 1913, *Geriatrics: Geriatric Medicine* was published in New York by Ignasz Nascher, a physician from Vienna. The book defined the need for a specialty dedicated to the needs of the elderly, just as the new specialty of pediatrics was beginning to focus on children. Nascher's principles are thoroughly consistent with the principles of modern geriatric medicine.

What makes a geriatrician different from an internist, family physician, or other specialist is not only a deeper knowledge of the kinds of illnesses that affect older people but also a scientific understanding of biological aging and how the social environment affects health as one ages. The geriatrician is much more likely to be able to answer a patient's question, "Is this what I can expect from old age, or is this a treatable condition?" As baby boomers age, this question will be asked more and more often, and the answer will define the aging experiences of millions of people. Further, finding the correct answer to this question is the only ethical way to contain health-care costs for the aging; it allows us to restrain demand for treatments that are ineffective and unnecessary while advocating for treatments that improve quality of life and function.

Aging in itself is not a disease, but illness and disability become more likely with advancing age. The goals of geriatric medicine are not simply to diagnose and treat specific diseases or specific organ system failures but rather to take into account the patient's physical and mental condition, and, equally important, the patient's own values and priorities. At least 50 percent of older people suffer from multiple chronic conditions that require coordination among several specialties. The geriatrician calls on specialists when needed but also coordinates care to avoid ordering redundant tests and treatments and facilitates communication between the specialists. Geriatricians also assist with the important transitions between home, hospital, nursing home, assisted living, and rehabilitation center that often characterize care for the elderly.

Numerous countries have adopted geriatric medicine. It came late to the United States. Despite Nascher's pioneering work, fellowship training programs in geriatric medicine began at VA hospitals only in the late 1970s and early 1980s. By the late 1980s, a board certification exam recognized additional qualifications in geriatrics for physicians certified in internal medicine, family medicine, and psychiatry.

The number of physicians receiving geriatric training has remained quite small, even though government reports have called for increasing expertise in geriatric medicine to guide the provision of appropriate and effective care for the growing older population. Currently, only three of the 125 medical schools in the United States have departments of geriatrics. In contrast, every medical school in Great Britain and 20 percent of those in Japan have such departments.

Moreover, less than half of the medical schools in the United States offer any comprehensive training program in geriatrics; and even in those that do, many medical students are not trained to care for the complex medical and social needs of older patients. There are only a few thousand board-certified geriatricians in the United States today, and the Alliance for Aging Research estimates that only about six hundred of those have had adequate formal training to teach and lead programs in medical schools.[2] Geriatricians are necessary not only to care for the most complex needs of older people but also, and perhaps more important, to ensure that all physicians—surgeons, internists, family physicians, psychiatrists, and others—have a basic knowledge of the fundamental principles of the science of aging and geriatric medicine. We do not have nearly enough geriatricians to be the teachers, much less to provide the care that is needed.

Why don't more young people go into geriatric medicine? One reason is the negative attitudes about aging that characterize our society. To change these attitudes, we need role models who treat older people with respect and understand that improving the quality of life for older people is extremely gratifying work. Even with good teachers, however, Medicare's payment system for coordinating services (sometimes known as "cognitive services") has a chilling effect on the interest of young physicians going into geriatrics. Students leaving medical school, who may owe more than a hundred thousand dollars in educational loans, may be more attracted to specialties that focus on highly-paid procedures than to the equally demanding but much lower-paid specialty of coordinating care for older people.

The evolution of geriatric medicine provides a model for the kind of medical care that Medicare in the twenty-first century ought to embrace. The specialty includes two basic features: a modern scientific understanding of the biology of aging, along with a humanistic and holistic approach to treating older patients; and an interdisciplinary commitment to manage complex care, to anticipate and avoid complications, coordinate multiple specialty providers, and seek functional approaches to goals rather than focusing only on laboratory values or disease-oriented medical treatment.

Today's Medicare is built on a model defined by the terms of medical insurance as understood in 1965. Little understanding of aging populations and no awareness of geriatric medicine went into its design. Most of the recent efforts to reform Medicare have focused on finances and the details of insurance coverage, which only perpetuate the original mistakes in the program's perspective. The overarching mission should be to meet the needs of the growing population of older people in the United States and respond to the promise of longevity for all of us. This is where Medicare needs radical changes. Establishing this priority is the challenge of this book.

Of course, finding our way involves evaluating finances and the extent of coverage, and avoiding breaking the bank. The practical features of Medicare policy affect everyone, and here rises the second order of Medicare's potential: that we forge a stronger social contract and intergenerational ties that are transparent and just, regardless of the details or directions we happen to choose.

A FASCINATING CASE

Medical trainees are taught to seek out unusual disorders that need aggressive intervention so that they can learn about exotic diseases and get practice in the use of medical technology. As a newly certified specialist in geriatric medicine, I found that this orientation led doctors to overlook the most obvious areas of need. Many older people were coming to the hospital with very common disorders not always needing technological intervention but often needing care.

It was difficult to convince the young physicians in training—the interns, residents, and medical students—that these elderly patients were interesting. One such case was a ninety-three-year old man with severe dementia and urinary incontinence. His wife brought him into the emergency room with a chief complaint of "unable to get out of bed."

When the house staff asked the wife how long her husband had been in this condition, she said, "For months." Why had she brought him in today? She said her daughter, who normally helped look after him, had taken ill and was in the hospital. The wife, who was frail herself, could not take care of the old man on her own.

To most emergency-room physicians, this kind of a case is known as a "dump." Even worse, the man might be referred to as a "Gomer," which stands for "get out of my emergency room." My job was to convince young doctors that this was instead a fascinating case.

What makes a patient interesting is usually a rare disease or a diagnostic puzzle with unusual signs. In treating this man, we discovered a number of important medical issues. Although he had an underlying diagnosis of Alzheimer's disease, his mental condition had become much worse after he developed a urinary tract infection (this can happen with any infection); the infection also led to urinary incontinence. Both conditions made it much harder for his wife to take care of him at home. Further, several weeks in bed had led to muscle atrophy and loss of strength, leaving him unable to stand upright.

A number of these conditions were reversible. On admission to the hospital, with treatment of his urinary tract infection and better hydration, the man's level of awareness improved. He was able to recognize his wife, although his memory remained significantly impaired. After ten days of physical therapy, he was able to sit upright and stand for short periods of time without blacking out.

This was perhaps not the dramatic cure that the young doctors were looking for, but it made it possible for this man to go home with his wife rather than to a nursing home. This was a critical accomplishment. Millions of patients with similar conditions are not served so well, and they and their families are left feeling abandoned and frustrated by the modern health-care system. Too often medical solutions apply technology to a physical diagnosis and deem areas less susceptible to technical or pharmaceutical intervention as "social problems." This perspective fails to recognize the patient's point of view in the concept of health and greatly reduces the efficacy of medicine.

Coming of Age

For many older Americans and their families, medical advances have only widened the gap between economic resources and available care. Older citizens face similar or worse financial obstacles to health care today than in 1965. Studies of household finances in the years before Medicare showed that medical care for older adults imposed significant costs, which often had to be borne by their children.[3] The elderly, with an income only half that of the general population, faced higher health-care costs. According to health surveys at the time, people aged sixty-five and over were twice as likely as others to be chronically ill and were hospitalized for twice as long. Medical costs were high, and only half of the older adult population had insurance. Single or widowed women were likely to have significantly fewer of their hospital costs covered by insurance.[4]

In 1958 older people reported spending more than double what younger people spent on their health care each year. As age increased, income decreased and health declined, making it even harder to pay medical bills. In 1962 only 38 percent of retired Americans had health insurance. Data from the National Health Survey for the years 1958 through 1960 show that half of the elderly's short hospital stays were not covered by health insurance. Even so, older adults with insurance used about two and a half times as much hospital care as uninsured older adults, indicating a positive correlation between availability of insurance and health-care use. In other words, older people without insurance were probably not seeking care when they genuinely needed it.[5]

Reaching age sixty-five often made health insurance too costly to purchase, and hospitalization commonly caused people to incur large debts. The Health Insurance Plan of Greater New York reported the impact:

We have many enrollees who, upon attainment of age 65, become ineligible to continue group enrollment and no longer have part or all of their premium paid by an employer or welfare fund. Two out of three of these people drop their health insurance. They simply cannot afford to go on, at a time when their income is reduced, to pick up the full cost of health insurance which previously had been paid for all or in part by the employers. This is really tragic.[6]

At the same time, there was widespread recognition that private sector insurance would not be able to remedy the situation. In 1964 a Blue Cross spokesman testified before Congress that "insuring everyone over age sixty-five is a losing business that must be subsidized."[7]

Since then, Medicare has become popular among beneficiaries, a major source of payment to doctors and hospitals, and the focus of concern over growing expenditures. Many changes have been instituted to add benefits and contain rising costs. These changes have been piecemeal, instituted by Congress in concert with lobbyists for major interest groups, like doctors, hospitals, drug companies, and insurance companies. Significant policy interventions, such as the prospective-payment system with diagnosis-related groups (DRGs), instituted in 1984, undoubtedly changed patterns of consumption, especially by shortening the length of hospital stays; but none of them managed to hold down the rate of growth in expenditures per person or to create a truly effective health-care system that reflects the principles of modern geriatric medicine.

In the last forty years biomedical technology has expanded tremendously, offering us an array of new and expensive options for care. Health care has evolved into a corporate enterprise worth more than a trillion dollars per year, or more than 14 percent of the value of all goods and services in the United States. With annual expenditures of more than $260 billion, Medicare is commonly viewed as a significant driver of the system. Medicare's impending financial doom could prompt changes. Powerful stakeholders have come to expect high incomes and high returns on investment. In some senses, these pressures freeze the system into a preference for the status quo. Policy makers will certainly face growing pressure to deliver a program that is affordable, effective, and efficient.

Medicare coverage of acute care has improved the health of older adults in the United States. It has lightened the financial burden on the elderly and their families, and it has extended lives and improved quality of life. Yet despite these successes, Medicare is a clumsy, heavily bureaucratic program that relies on Congressional debate to make medical adjustments for almost forty million people with very different health-care needs.

ADJUSTING TO LONGEVITY

Access to modern medical technology has made only a small contribution to the gift of increasing longevity we have experienced over the last fifty years. Environmental and social factors have stronger effects on healthy aging than medical treatments do. Far from contributing to longevity, medicine is facing a new challenge for which it is largely unprepared. As the number and proportion of older people in the population continue to increase, a satisfactory solution to the problem of paying for adequate medical care for the aged will become even more important.

Today's Medicare still does not address the growing importance of self-care, chronic care, and low-technology approaches to supporting quality of life and reducing suffering at the end of life. These approaches to care are based on interdisciplinary collaboration between nursing, social work, and other helping professionals. Investments in these areas have been much lower than in other technology-based areas, such as medical equipment, which Medicare has helped to define and perpetuate.

Traditional insurance carriers, including Medicare, do not cover coordinated team-based care. Innovation to increase value in medical practice is stifled by rigid payment categories. Many analysts believe a major cause of the rising costs of Medicare is the use of unnecessary or inappropriate expensive medical technology because Medicare creates financial incentives for high-tech interventions rather than personalized problem-solving.

Policy makers have an opportunity to design a comprehensive program that incorporates neglected areas, such as long-term care, into a system of true health security for the aging population. This requires first a change in thinking.

FUNDING CHALLENGES

Integrating geriatric medicine into Medicare reform is primarily a responsibility of the health-care professions. Clearly, however, enduring innovation will not be possible without an appropriate environment of financial incentives. Of greatest concern at present is the projected depletion of the Part A Hospital Insurance (HI) trust fund, which is funded by the Federal Insurance Contributions Act (FICA) payroll tax of 4.9 percent, split evenly between employers and employees. Part A pays for care in hospitals, skilled nursing facilities, and hospices. With a focus on fiscal crisis and a command to remain budget-neutral, reformers are looking more toward incrementally adjusting benefits and deductibles, like a commercial insurer, than toward organizing to fulfill a vital public mandate.

In 1997, HI trustees forecasted that funds would be depleted as early as 2001. Passage of the Balanced Budget Act (BBA) of 1997 reduced provider reimbursements and funds dedicated to graduate medical education; as a result, the financial picture for the Medicare program improved considerably by 2000, but at great cost to providers. Care providers and academic medical centers protested enough to have some of the harsher measures of BBA moderated or delayed in the Balanced Budget Reconciliation Act (BBRA) of 1999.

With a booming economy and lower increases in health-care costs during the last years of the 1990s, HI solvency was projected to last until 2023. HI income exceeded expenditures by $4.8 billion in 1998 and by $21 billion in 1999, yielding the first trust-fund surpluses since 1994.[8] The drastic tax cuts and national deficits since 2000 raise concerns that Medicare HI shortages will arrive sooner than 2023. The political calculus seems to rule out any possibility of increases in FICA taxes, even though such contributions would amount to far less than most families are paying out of pocket for health care.

About 2010, when the oldest baby boomers begin to reach age sixty-five, there is expected to be a ratio of 3.6 workers to each Medicare beneficiary. By the time the youngest boomers turn sixty-five in 2030, the ratio is estimated to be only 2.3 workers per beneficiary. As life expectancy continues to increase, the ratio is expected to decline even further.[9] The Medicare Prescription Drug Improvement and Modernization Act of 2003 attempts to address escalating costs by creating incentives for more private-sector participation through various private plans. For example, private plans are paid at a higher rate than traditional fee-for-service Medicare and are allowed to negotiate better rates for drug coverage.

This effort to push Medicare recipients into managed care might be viewed as a breach of the fundamental social commitment of Medicare, a thrust to impose a free-enterprise ideology that aims to reduce costs without evidence that it would improve care.

The Social Contract

The proper role of government in providing basic social services is a question that continues to elicit deep ambivalence. The nation appears unwilling to provide universal health insurance for all citizens—or even for all children—yet we rely on government at every level to guarantee many other fundamental features of civilized society. In health care, the vision of what we are trying to achieve is too often obscure or missing all together.

A positive aging society requires a strong national commitment to the social-insurance foundation of Medicare. Without modern, affordable, flexible health-care insurance for older citizens, U.S. society could turn into a world where old age is a feared condition burdensome to families. The continued success of our aging society depends on our understanding the benefits of a sound social contract for all of us. My chances of successful aging depend on the collective goods of a productive society—and so do yours.

With dramatic successes that allow people to expect to live to a considerable age, modern medicine has become much like public health in its relevance to social well-being and its dependence on a viable social contract. All of us want to drink uncontaminated water and eat safe food. We understand that the government has an important role in protecting us from infectious agents, whether they are indigenous, manufactured by industry, or, more improbably, introduced by terrorists.

The aging of society has made medical care a similarly valuable social commodity. Given the unpredictability of health needs, it is impossible for individuals or families to plan for and fund their own health care. This situation requires a wide sharing of risk across a large population. Medicare accomplishes this goal admirably. Any changes to Medicare that lead to more individual risk will do irreparable damage to the fundamental strength of social insurance. Society will suffer if older people are put at risk and not allowed to participate productively and actively in it. Keeping older people active through basic health care is good for business, good for cultural and social life, and good for family solidarity.

In all the debate about what to do with Medicare, we too often lose sight of the successes of the program. Medicare is partly responsible for the increased health of today's older adults, and also helps to insulate them from financial ruin, but benefits accrue to others besides the old folks. Medicare insulates whole families from the risks and burdens of health-care expenses for aging parents that would otherwise absorb the resources of a younger generation. Families are able to invest in other things.

Partisan political posturing is making it increasingly difficult to meet this broad social goal. Policy in Washington often reflects ideology, advancing ideas about privatization at the expense of objectives for health security. Energetic lobbying by various health-care industry stakeholders adds support for partisan interests. Impatience with such divisive politics is growing. We have come to understand more clearly why our health-care system, the most costly in the world, has been unable to provide safe and effective care to patients. New approaches to improving the quality of care are appearing everywhere, linking purchasers, consumers, and providers as well as academics, public officials, and communities in a rising crescendo of concern and effort.

As the largest insurer in the country, Medicare has a vital interest in the quality of health care. The program's ability to help maintain it will be fundamentally harmed without a sense of the social contract, recognizing a public commitment to the success of health security. The new promise of successful aging forces us to contemplate sweeping changes in health-care organization to facilitate geriatric medicine and to establish efficient forms of payment to support it.

Principal Points

If Medicare encouraged the delivery of high-quality primary geriatric care, more Americans would age productively and be able to stay active and involved in our communities. As the aging baby boomers and their families struggle with critical decisions about how to reshape Medicare for the twenty-first century, the following points merit consideration:

- Medicare influences the longevity, welfare, and productivity of older adults. All of society stands to benefit from the program. The financial risks of providing adequate health security are too great to be borne by competing insurance carriers or by individual families. The strength of the social contract justifying Medicare is the primary attribute the program must maintain.

- Medicare needs to modernize and promote widespread access to advances that allow older adults to benefit from the early and active management of chronic illness. Decreasing age-related functional decline and disability should be the major health policy goal of the twenty-first century.

- Medicare's payment structure should encourage the practice of the highest-quality geriatric medicine. An adequately financed system, without the overuse distortion of fee for service, would reward providers who follow the principles of modern geriatric medicine.

- Good models of successful care management for older adults do exist and should serve as instructive models for Medicare.

- Outpatient prescription drugs are an essential part of modern geriatric medicine and should be covered by Medicare in an evidence-based, cost-effective manner.

· Medicare should expand its hospice benefit to address diverse end-of-life needs.

Professionals and the Public

Health care is a dynamic field of activity in which we all have an interest. Solvency will always be a challenge as we face continuous medical innovation and rising expectations. No insurance plan can or should cover all possible medical tests and treatments, but we do expect insurance coverage to keep up with effective new treatments. We would also like to avoid rationing necessary treatment, especially if such rationing results in prejudicial distinctions between people or practices. Moreover, we should expect Medicare to cover comprehensive, patient-centered care for chronic illness to reduce the caregiving burden on families and enhance function, quality of life, and dignity for those with disabilities.

New developments in pharmacology, genomics, and various aspects of medical technology are truly compelling, and there is no reason not to take advantage of them—except cost. Eventually we need to take a hard look at the value of such innovations and decide how to distribute our resources efficiently. A working market usually accomplishes this for us; but in health care, the market is constrained from operating freely.

Preserving lives with new, high-tech solutions is an area in which American medicine excels and of which we are rightly proud. We should be equally enthusiastic about saving lives among those who now fall through the gaps in the system, often for simple reasons that health-care professionals can resolve with low-tech compassion and attention to service. This is a vast area of undeveloped territory. Exciting developments in acute care tend to overshadow the chronic health-care needs of a much larger part of the population. Implementing comprehensive geriatric medicine among the population most likely to benefit from it requires a new focus and redirection of resources.

Everyone who works in the health professions has felt challenged by the pressures of the competitive market environment. Physicians can feel helpless, manipulated, and unable to meet the needs of their patients. This feeling has been reinforced by data about shortfalls and problems in quality of care. The principles of modern geriatric medicine would put the health-care provider team back at the center of health-care decision making, rather than in the position of following arbitrary, bureaucratic rules about which treatments and services are covered by insurance. Supported by evidence-based practice, professionals with clinical expertise and knowledge of the individual patient and family should be the ones making decisions about medical necessity. The only way this change can happen is through a broad-based population focus, with the purchasers of health care invested in the long-term health security of the whole population.

Of course, our goal as a society ought to be health-care coverage for everyone, not just for the elderly. In 1965, Medicare was viewed as a first step toward national health insurance. Forty years later, the demand for a model system remains unmet, and a fresh start appears possible. The *Journal of the American Medical Association* of August 13, 2003, featured a statement signed by about eight thousand physicians that endorsed single-payer national health insurance.[10] Actual prospects for the plan are perhaps as unpromising as ever, but clearly the kind of dialogue about health-care reform common a decade ago is being resumed with determination.

Opinions differ about the correct approach to universal health coverage, but a couple of points are immediately clear. First, broad-based social insurance with a large and diverse risk pool is the only plausible solution. Without it, the people with the greatest needs tend to be excluded and face prohibitive insurance premiums and out-of-pocket costs. Insurance companies are motivated to avoid offering coverage to unhealthy people and have learned to identify risks and concentrate on the 70 to 90 percent of the population with lower-than-average health-care expenses. Public and charity programs are left with the responsibility for the greatest portion of total personal health-care expenditures among a small segment of the population. The segmentation of risk and costs is impossible to sustain. If everyone were enrolled in a universal health-care system, the problem would disappear.

Second, a universal health-care system with a single source of payment that can be managed electronically is much more efficient. Medicare administers one of the most efficient payment systems for health insurance in the world and may be reasonably viewed as a model for a universal system. By that standard, overhead and administrative costs could be reduced from the current 15 to 20 percent typical of commercial insurers to about 3 to 5 percent.

Expanding health insurance beyond Medicare to cover everyone in society, starting with children, should be a priority in the United States, and our approach should be informed by our experience with Medicare. A society that is good to grow old in is a society that is good for everyone. That valuable lesson in the social contract supports our quest for greater enfranchisement. For all of us, Medicare matters.

So this book is not just about elderly and disabled people in need of health care, nor is it addressed solely to Medicare policy wonks. It touches on issues of vital interest to all of us: to anyone who has a parent or grandparent, who expects to grow old with dignity, and who cares about maintaining the productivity and vitality of our society.

CHAPTER 2

Longevity and Health

What makes the Man of the Year unique? . . . He has a sense
of economic security unmatched in history. Granted an ever-
lengthening adolescence and lifespan, he no longer feels the
cold pressures of hunger and mortality. . . . Science and the
knowledge explosion have armed him with more tools to
choose his life pattern than he can always use: physical and
intellectual mobility, personal and financial opportunity, a vista
of change accelerating in every direction. Untold adventures
await him. He is the man who will land on the moon, cure
cancer and the common cold, lay out blight-proof, smog-free
cities, enrich the underdeveloped world, and, no doubt, write
finis to poverty and war.

> *Time* magazine, "Man of the Year 1966:
> The Man—and Woman—of 25 and Under"

Baby boomers have been a potent social force all their lives. Born during
the period of postwar affluence from 1946 to 1964, their large numbers
required the expansion of public schools. As young adults they defined
what it meant to be young and created a counterculture so powerful it
rocked the status quo. As middle-aged parents, they have changed the
character of American families with higher divorce rates, increased workforce participation by women, and varied family structures. Their influence on how we think about aging is likely to be just as powerful.

When *Time* celebrated the baby boomers as Man and Woman of the
Year in 1966, the magazine claimed for them the opportunity to live long,

healthy, and successful lives. They had the advantages of science and modernity. They also had the advantage of numbers—the potential as a large, influential group to create a society in which it would be possible to enjoy growing old. As the boomers age, however, their numbers are less celebrated than they once were: indeed, it sometimes sounds as though they are becoming a threat to national security. A journalist writing that all seventy-six million boomers will have reached the age of sixty-five by 2030 is now more likely to be concerned about the effect on the federal budget than about the scientific, medical, or social innovations that will help this cohort age well.

Why are we so afraid of an aging society? For one thing, the dramatic demographic shifts currently occurring are unprecedented in human history. Although the aging of society is now a common topic, we have not yet adapted our public policy or collective psyche to meet it. In general, American culture is steeped in negative stereotypes of aging: older adults are portrayed as dependent, irrelevant, incapable, and out of touch. Such images may become a self-fulfilling prophecy. Although the average American life span is now seventy-six years, meaning that many live far beyond that age, we still expect people to retire at age sixty-five or earlier. Early retirement helps create a bifurcated society in which younger people and older people live in separate worlds, rarely seeing one another in their daily routines. Likewise, the popularity of retirement communities, combined with the mobility of American families, makes intergenerational housing uncommon. Missing opportunities to befriend people of different generations, even within families, impoverishes everyone.

The financial implications of an aging society also make us uneasy. Social Security and Medicare form the largest nondiscretionary components of the federal budget. The entitlement nature of these two programs has always been vulnerable to ideological attack, the more so now that projected budget deficits reinforce a sense of crisis. It is difficult to focus on social change that promotes successful aging when sound bites arouse fears that extending life expectancy will undermine the economic vitality of our society.

Older people need more health care than young people. As scientific and medical advances enable us to prolong and improve life, health-care costs will continue to increase. If we do not improve the way our society deals with its older adults, embrace the success of longevity, and enhance its productivity, then there will be a real cause for concern. We have the capacity to make longevity a blessing for most people and less of a crisis for many more. Our goals should include the use of modern medicine in a more coordinated, efficient, and humane system than exists today; restructuring expectations about work as we age; and an informed public, able to guide political choices in the complex network of modern health care. The eminent gerontologist Bernice Neugarten once said, "A society that is good for older people is good for everyone."

The boomer generation represents a unique resource for crafting new solutions to perceived social problems. The boomers may not have wiped out war or poverty, but they have revolutionized many aspects of the world, such as science, business, and global communication. Although they represent diverse ideological viewpoints, during their lifetimes the United States has seen an overall strengthening of community relations, social tolerance, and human and civil rights. If the vitality of democratic government persists, boomers in the coming decades may once again prove their role as innovators, showing us that an aging America is really a success story and longevity the sign of a flourishing civilization.

Successful Aging

Never before have so many people lived to a healthy old age. In the forty-five hundred years from the Bronze Age to the year 1900, life expectancy is estimated to have increased twenty-seven years. Between 1900 and 1990, life expectancy increased by at least that much again. Of all the people who have ever lived to be sixty-five years old, half are estimated to be alive today.[1]

In 1900 there were about 3 million people aged sixty-five and over in the United States, making up 4.1 percent of the population.[2] By 1963 the number had grown to 17.5 million; and one could reasonably expect to survive to old age. This demographic news sparked interest in Washington, where Medicare policy was born. In 2000 about 35 million citizens were aged sixty-five and over, constituting 12.5 percent of the population. By 2030, this age group will account for about 70 million people, or 20 percent of the population.

Eighty percent of Americans now survive to age sixty-five, double the percentage at the turn of the century. Life expectancy at age sixty-five is now seventeen years, five years longer than at the turn of the century. Many sixty-five-year-olds remain physically and mentally active and capable of contributing to society on many levels.

Those over age eighty-five, known as the oldest old, are the fastest-growing segment of the population. In 1900, they accounted for only 4 percent of all people over age sixty-five. Now that figure is 12 percent and growing; it is expected to triple by 2040 to 14.3 million.[3]

Even living to one hundred is no longer a rarity. In 1950, there were roughly 3,000 centenarians in the United States. In 2000, centenarians on the rolls of the Social Security Administration numbered about 65,000. In 2010, estimates put the number at well over 100,000, perhaps as high as 200,000. In fifty years the figure may approach 1 million. Some authorities talk seriously of life expectancies of 110 or 120 years and anticipate someday reaching 150.[4] Interestingly, about 90 percent of centenarians are women.[5] We do not fully understand this survival advantage of women, but the fact may be important for shaping public policy as the number of the oldest old continues to grow.

Although population projections are not always accurate, clearly we are witnessing a dramatic leap in life expectancy. We are living longer for a variety of medical, behavioral, and social reasons. In the first half of the twentieth century, improvements in public health were the main cause of increased life expectancy. Premature deaths, particularly among children, were greatly reduced. During that time, the United States improved sanitation, implemented occupational-health policies, passed child labor laws, relieved residential overcrowding, and improved the safety and purity of food and water. Better education, resulting from the establishment of public schools and mandatory attendance policies, is also linked with the increase in life expectancy.

In the second half of the twentieth century, dramatic increases in life expectancy have continued, especially for older people, as medical science has developed the ability to cure, control, or prevent once-fatal diseases. Antibiotics work against life-threatening infections, which were formerly the leading cause of death. Insulin can control diabetes. Advances in anesthesia and surgical techniques help us to treat cancer, cardiovascular disease, and bone, joint, and even brain and spinal-cord disorders. Risk factors for illness are understood better: we recognize that treatment for hypertension can prevent stroke and reducing blood lipids can prevent heart attacks. More attention is being paid to behavioral risks like smoking, physical inactivity, obesity, and unhealthy eating. Screening for early detection of disease is more common, especially for cancers, and it is accompanied by better treatments. Medical technology enables people to survive previously fatal diseases. Hospital intensive-care units make it possible to effectively treat pneumonia and heart attacks, which, until recently, were usually fatal events for those seventy or older.

Despite this array of medical advances, the overall incidence rates of the three leading causes of death in the United States—heart disease, cancer, and stroke—are much the same today as they were in 1965. We are not preventing these diseases as much as postponing them. A heart attack now occurs more commonly after age sixty-five than before, but it remains a leading cause of death. People are surviving once-fatal infections and other diseases that are now curable and end up living long enough to experience age-related illnesses. That many will eventually experience heart disease, cancer, or stroke can be attributed to the simple fact of longevity. Delaying disease onset represents significant progress, but truly preventing these life-threatening events is biologically unlikely.

The definition of premature death depends on circumstances and personal values. If we could establish a normal life expectancy, then the idea of a premature death would be defined as someone dying before that time; but chronological age is not the only factor in this determination. Increasingly, premature death will be defined in terms of quality of life rather than number of years.

Consider two scenarios. If a healthy, vigorous eighty-year-old attorney who still practices law contracts pneumonia and dies, his death is likely to be viewed as premature. With adequate medical care to treat the pneumonia or prevent it through appropriate immunizations and access to primary care, the man might have lived another ten to twenty years with a reasonable expectation of an acceptable quality of life. On the other hand, the death of an eighty-year-old man in the late stages of Alzheimer's disease, living in a nursing home, unable to recognize any family members, bedridden, and unable to feed himself, might be viewed as a blessing and an end to suffering. Aggressive and intrusive measures to treat his pneumonia, such as putting him on a ventilator in an intensive-care unit, would be regarded as unseemly and possibly even unethical. Yet the same approach to treat the active lawyer would be considered appropriate care.

Medicare's promise of universal access to health care for all beneficiaries has improved the health and increased the longevity of older Americans. The availability of Medicare reimbursement has encouraged the development and common use of many of the medical advances that enable the baby boomers to look forward to an active old age. Without Medicare payment, medical innovation might have been stifled, and today's newest medical technologies would not exist.

Remarkable advances in modern science are prompting us to change the way we think about aging. Tomorrow's medical discoveries could further change views of aging and the kind of health-care coverage people will need. Despite Medicare's enormous success at increasing longevity and improving access to health care, change is needed to ensure that society can continue to provide older Americans with access to the highest-quality health care.

Aging Research

Aging research, once a backwater of biology, is now a hot topic for both scientists and the general public. Magazines and newspapers aimed at both scientific and lay audiences have special columns and issues dedicated to aging news. In September 2000 *Scientific American* dedicated an entire issue to "the quest to beat aging," covering research aimed at increasing longevity and suggesting the ultimate goal of immortality. Most aging research is aimed at the more prosaic goals of delaying and treating age-related illnesses and improving the quality of life for those with diseases we do not yet know how to prevent.

The recent surge of interest in aging research can be attributed to three factors. First, the baby boomers are now the aging generation. For better or worse, those in this generation have repeatedly demanded attention and made things happen, creating new products and forming new social movements to satisfy their needs through each stage of life. As a group, we should not expect baby boomers to "go gentle into that good night."

Second, many boomers face the logistical and financial challenges of caring for their aging parents.[6] Issues facing family caregivers are being pushed to the forefront of national attention. Congress passed legislation in 2000 to establish the National Family Caregiver Support Program, which gives funds to state offices for the aging in order to provide family caregivers with information, assistance, counseling, training, and respite care. Although the program will not be able to meet all the needs of families struggling to take care of frail relatives at home, it signifies public concern and incremental progress toward a solution.

Third, aging research is popular because of the dramatic advances of medical science. Medical research in the 1960s and 1970s focused on age-related issues similar to those in the news today, studying osteoporosis, cardiovascular disease, cancer, and other age-related diseases; but recent advances in molecular and genetic science are radically changing the character of all biomedical research, leading to potentially dramatic advances in prevention as well as treatment. New knowledge of the biochemical, molecular, and genetic processes has further changed the way we think about aging. The implications are profound for improving quality of life—and for increasing medical costs.

A complex web of factors influences aging. Genetic and hereditary factors, the environment, socioeconomic status, stressors, disease processes, and diet all play important roles. We are beginning to question whether aging is a sum of diseases, essentially an accumulation of wear and tear on the body over time, or a genetically predetermined, biological event much like embryonic development, sexual maturation, or menopause. It most likely involves both of these processes—progressive wear and tear as well as some genetically programmed events. The processes are probably also interrelated. For example, some genes probably help the body repair cellular and tissue damage; and other genes may govern the metabolic changes that occur during aging, allowing alteration of the aging "clock" itself.[7]

Cells in our bodies are stressed over the course of a lifetime and eventually become less capable of responding to injury. Damage accumulates. Various other functions performed by cells also decline over time. Mitochondria, the energy-producing components of our cells, exhibit slower metabolic processes over time.[8] Cells synthesize fewer proteins, enzymes, and chemical signals.

Our improved knowledge of basic science has increased the sophistication of the questions researchers now ask. Several key principles underlie these advances. First, we know that the cells that make up human tissues and organs—including cells for the immune system, blood, skeletal system, skin, and brain—participate in a vast network of intercommunication. Through complex signaling systems, cells can communicate a wide variety of messages: when to mature, when to multiply, when to synthesize other chemical signals, even when to migrate to other parts of the body. Can we discover the signals that lead to the aging of cells or tissues? And can we use these cues to our advantage? Taking the inquiry a step further, genetic information contained in cells may help us determine how and when we age. What are the coded genetic messages contained in cells? Can we work from a genetic perspective to prolong certain stages and forestall others?

Scientific medical advances have already allowed us to redefine and change the course of many diseases of old age. Researchers have reexamined cognitive impairment, the weakening of the immune system, and musculoskeletal disorders such as arthritis and osteoporosis, and these conditions are now recognized as treatable. In some cases, we have already begun to use new technology to develop specific treatments, such as hip and knee replacements. In other cases, researchers are beginning to plot the specific mechanisms of disease. Recent successes for Alzheimer's disease, for example, could eventually lead to an effective treatment.

In addition, population studies and clinical trials have shown us that many of the disabling diseases of aging can be slowed or avoided by behavioral changes. Exercising regularly, eating a healthy diet, controlling weight, and staying active mentally and physically are all demonstrably beneficial. These practices will be vital to the healthy aging of the baby boomers.

Policy makers might be tempted to conclude that all health problems are self-induced and that better efforts at prevention will reduce the overall need for Medicare spending; but this is not true, for two big reasons. First, most medical conditions of aging are not prevented by even the healthiest lifestyles: these include Alzheimer's and Parkinson's disease, osteoarthritis and osteoporosis, and most cancers. Second, medical interventions may be essential to keep people active. Artificial joints make it easier to maintain physical activity; hearing aids, cochlear implants, and cataract surgery can be important in maintaining mental and social activities. Prevention is critical to successful aging, but biomedical science is an increasingly vital partner in prevention.

Following are a few examples of the kinds of age-related conditions and accompanying scientific advances that will be significant concerns in geriatric medicine and in Medicare's future.

BONES AND JOINTS: OSTEOPOROSIS AND ARTHRITIS

Osteoporosis and arthritis are common complaints of aging that can be extremely painful and debilitating. Both used to be considered a part of normal aging rather than preventable or treatable diseases. New knowledge of the processes involved in progressive tissue damage and decline has prompted researchers to look for ways to counteract it. Can we engineer tissues for the skeleton that can halt or reverse age-related degenerative change? Scientists have proposed mechanisms, including the use of gene transfer, creating new tissues with stem cells (embryonic cells that have not yet differentiated into specific tissues), and genetically engineered signaling molecules to enhance bone formation. Other proposed methods include creating a molecular carrier that would deliver signals, or even cells themselves, to the sites where repair is needed.[9]

Osteoporosis, a progressive loss of bone density more common in older women than men, can lead to disability and a high risk of dependency or death as a result of hip and vertebral fractures. A number of promising advances in this field may slow or prevent the condition. Hormone replacement therapy is demonstrably effective, but new information suggests that it can double the risk of heart disease and may increase the risk of breast cancer. More recent medications that prevent bone demineralization are becoming available, and more are under development that may substantially delay or prevent this disabling condition.

JOINT REPLACEMENT

Arthritis, usually in the form of osteoarthritis, is the most commonly reported chronic condition among those aged sixty-five and over. Half of the elderly are affected and many are seriously disabled by it. Lost productivity from arthritis-related disability has been estimated at 1 percent of the U.S. gross national product.[10] Arthritis also prevents exercise and physical activity known to be associated with healthier aging.

Drug treatment for osteoarthritis decreases disability and improves functional independence, but consistent high doses of anti-inflammatory medications require close management to avoid complications such as internal bleeding, renal failure, or heart problems. When medication is not enough, several effective surgical treatments are available. Hip and knee replacements are a common and highly successful form of arthritis treatment.

Serious complications associated with inactivity, including osteoporosis, muscle weakness, falls, heart disease, and depression, can be ameliorated by restoring activity. Cartilage replacement, natural or artificial, is a promising possibility that is less surgically intensive than total joint replacement. Over the next several decades, interventions through drugs and surgery are likely to become more common for osteoarthritis, diminishing its disabling effects among greater numbers of the elderly.[11]

DESIGNER HORMONES

Changes in hormone levels during aging have a range of effects on the human body. Declining estrogen levels, for example, lead to loss of bone mass, increased risk of osteoporosis, and possibly other effects, such as a decline in certain aspects of brain function. As a result, some postmenopausal women use hormone replacement therapies to raise their estrogen levels. Indications of side effects, including an increased risk of breast cancer, is leading to the development of "designer" hormones—hormones synthesized in the laboratory in order to enhance positive and reduce negative effects. To avoid the risk of breast cancer, for example, a designer hormone could be engineered to target bone cells only, without affecting breast tissue.

Scientists are still investigating whether estrogen and other hormones protect brain function. If the idea is confirmed, then new hormone therapies could improve normal memory and delay or prevent the onset of Alzheimer's disease. Similarly, testosterone, growth hormone, and other naturally occurring substances may promote healthy aging. Current growth-hormone treatments tend to improve the feeling and appearance of fitness, but their clinical effectiveness is doubtful, and adverse effects are in some cases substantial.[12] Public enthusiasm for these treatments needs to be countered by caution from physicians, but hormone treatments of various kinds are certainly on the horizon.

ALZHEIMER'S DISEASE: COGNITIVE ENHANCERS

Cognitive impairment and memory loss related to Alzheimer's disease are among the most devastating conditions of aging. Overcoming these conditions could alleviate much of the fear of aging and dramatically change the way people think about the later stages of life. One promising area of research, while still in a very early stage, focuses on developing cognitive enhancers that interact directly with receptors in the temporal lobe—the brain's memory center.

Neuroscientists have discovered substances in the brain that might be related to Alzheimer's disease. Clinical trials have been conducted for numerous medications to interrupt the possible causes of brain cell damage and stimulate brain-cell activity to reduce or delay the cognitive impairments related to Alzheimer's disease. Some have been shown to slow but not reverse the progression of functional decline in Alzheimer's disease. Research in prevention is examining antioxidants, anti-inflammatory medications, and hormones. Drugs that enhance alertness may improve the common memory lapses of aging. Memory can also be enhanced by exercises like learning new skills or solving puzzles.

All of these potential treatments offer only limited results to date, but they illustrate an improved understanding of one of the most feared diseases of aging. New discoveries may relieve that fear. Prospects are good that Alzheimer's will be a treatable condition in the coming decades. In

addition, now that genes related to Alzheimer's disease have been identified, it may be possible to target treatments for different forms of the
disease.

CONTROLLING CELL LONGEVITY

Telomerase is an enzyme believed to govern chromosomal aging through
its protective action on telomeres, the outermost tips of the chromosome
arms. With each cell division, a small segment of telomeric DNA is lost.
Unless a cell has a constant supply, the gradual reduction of telomerase
signals the cell to stop dividing, and cell death occurs.

Scientists are hoping that supplying telomerase can help to prevent
various diseases. By helping "good" cells to survive, telomerase might be
used to counteract diseases that involve premature cell death, such as
macular degeneration, a disease that involves progressive cell death in the
retina. Macular degeneration is the most common cause of blindness in
older adults and as yet remains untreatable. Telomerase therapy could
also be used to initiate cell death in selected targets such as cancer cells.
In treating cancer, physicians would purposely inhibit telomerase in an
attempt to stop excessive cell division and initiate the death of cancer cells.

ANTIOXIDANT RESEARCH

Antioxidants have received much attention in the popular press for their
potential capacity to rein in dangerous "free radicals," unstable molecules
that can damage living cells and hasten senescence. Scientists are conducting research to determine if antioxidants (including vitamins C and
E) can halt the actions of scavenging free radicals. Thus far, success in the
laboratory has not been matched by significant clinical successes in humans, but public enthusiasm for anti-aging therapies is demonstrated in
the widespread popularity of over-the-counter antioxidants.

GENE THERAPY

Aging is a fundamental process that involves all biological systems, so it
is unlikely that discovery or modification of a single gene can affect the
entire aging process. Any therapy able to counteract or delay the aging
process would need to be multigenic and complex. Although gene therapy may not be the elusive fountain of youth, we are already beginning
to use new knowledge of genes to treat some diseases. Eventually, it

might be possible to use gene therapy to prevent or delay age-related disorders as well.

The Human Genome Project, begun in 1990, was designed to decode a representative example of the human genome by 2005. The project decoded the first human chromosome in December 1999 and completed mapping the genome in 2000, five years ahead of schedule. Making this knowledge therapeutically useful, however, involves locating pathways of biological function and also devising methods of administration once a target gene is identified.[13] Opinions vary widely as to how long it will take us to truly master the details.

Gene therapy is currently aimed at treating diseases that involve a specific defect in a sequence of DNA. Defects in DNA sequencing can cause genes to produce the wrong amount of protein or a faulty protein. Gene therapy replaces a defective gene with a normal one. New cancer treatments known as biotherapeutics, for example, use compounds made from proteins and genetic materials, and some involve gene therapy. The goals are to replace or repair damaged genes or boost the immune system.

Biotherapeutics has led to an explosion of new therapies. Currently, 350 drugs are in clinical trials for breast cancer alone.[14] Progress is being made in combating heart disease as well. Several companies are in a race to determine whether gene therapy and related techniques can be used to promote the development of new blood vessels in the heart, a process that might lead to a nonsurgical "self-bypass" around blocked coronary arteries.

Genetics research has already made it easier to identify who is at high risk for some specific diseases and may make it possible eventually to target prevention and detection technologies to the appropriate populations. Uncovering the complete genetic code will allow scientists to identify defective genes that could put individuals at higher risk of illness.[15] Using such knowledge for prevention would require matching genetic data to the population, a proposal that has already aroused passionate discussions about privacy rights.

The pace of progress varies greatly for different diseases. Gene-therapy trials are under way for diseases caused by a defect in a single gene, such as cystic fibrosis, but complex diseases involving multiple genes, such as breast cancer or Alzheimer's disease, will take longer to comprehend. Moreover, because environmental factors play an important role in the development of disease, modifying a gene will not always guarantee prevention or cure. Nevertheless, unraveling the mysteries of the gene promises to move us a giant step toward understanding, treating, and preventing age-related illness.

ORGAN TRANSPLANTATION

Organ transplantation can be highly effective, enabling patients to regain function without reliance on expensive and distressing long-term treatments, such as kidney dialysis. Many transplant procedures have become routine. We can replace kidneys, livers, hearts, lungs, pancreases, intestines, and corneas—and brain tissue, as in treatment for Parkinson's disease. Though costly, transplantation can add years of function to an individual's life, enhance quality of life, and reduce reliance on chronic care. Because the supply of donated organs currently cannot satisfy demand, waiting lists of potential recipients number in the tens of thousands, most of whom die before receiving a transplant. Understandably, this shortage has led to policies restricting eligibility for receiving a transplant, based on criteria such as the probable number of future life-years and other factors.

Although younger patients tend to be favored under this regime, over the past ten years this framework has begun to change. Transplant surgery has been highly successful for patients in their seventies and eighties, particularly for liver and heart transplants. Old age, once considered a prohibitive risk factor in transplant surgery, is no longer an adequate criterion for denial.[16] Improved, less toxic immunosuppression protocols help to increase the success rate of transplants. In older people, diminished immune functioning may in fact further reduce the risk of rejection of a new organ.[17]

One approach to meeting the organ shortage is xenotransplantation, using animal tissues or organs. Genetic manipulation can yield organs with a low likelihood of rejection. Pigs are the most commonly used animals because they have important genetic similarities to humans. Cardiac valve replacement surgery using pig valves has been successful for many years.[18] Xenografts of other tissues and whole organs could be extremely cost-effective and could become a common treatment option for a range of organ-failure diseases, but we must first overcome concerns about viruses originating in animal tissues—as some evidence suggests the HIV virus originated in primates—and also the so-called "yuck" factor associated with the idea of implanting animal tissue in humans.

Stem-cell research is another exciting direction in transplant science. Cells taken from very early embryos, consisting of four to eight cells, are often discarded during fertility treatments. These "undifferentiated pluripotential stem cells" can grow to become any organ or tissue in the body, depending on the molecular and hormonal signals they are given. Stem cells are capable of producing human tissues and organs for transplantation, thus avoiding the risk of animal viruses as well as the psychological aversion of the "yuck" factor.

Stem-cell research is conducted in many countries but is controversial in the United States because of religious objections. Some people believe that an embryo of even a few cells should be treated as a human being. Others point out that these embryos, created in the process of reproductive enhancement, can ethically be used for research since they would otherwise be discarded. Stem cells exist in tissues other than embryos, but research in these alternative directions is not well advanced. Scientists are confident the technical barriers to using alternative sources can be overcome, so stem cells may be eventually obtained without the use of embryos. It is not unrealistic to expect a surge of organ availability that will overcome the rationing regime and eliminate any justification for age-based restrictions on organ transplants.

DIABETES

Diabetes affects about 20 percent of those over sixty-five. Common complications include blindness, kidney failure, and neurological and circulatory problems that can lead to amputation of the lower extremities. Traditional management of elderly diabetics involves maintaining blood sugar levels slightly above normal, but this strategy has been found to exacerbate complications. New approaches demonstrate that tight blood sugar control can significantly delay the onset of disabling complications. Insulin analogues show improved delivery and greater stability.[19] Medication and careful management can promote better health.

The insulin pump, an implantable device that regulates blood-sugar levels, is a highly effective management tool.[20] The pump has been used primarily in younger patients, reflecting a presumption of inevitable decline among the elderly, but the technology could also substantially reduce diabetes-related morbidity in elderly patients. Another treatment, pancreatic beta-cell transplantation,[21] is currently in clinical trials and could potentially cure diabetes. Both new treatments can dramatically improve outcomes but require close management, often including intensive medical or nursing supervision and an interdisciplinary approach.[22]

HEART DISEASE

Heart disease is a major cause of disability and death among the elderly. The severity of the condition increases with age. A number of new treatments, including angioplasty, bypass surgery, and drug therapy, have improved and extended lives. These proven successes are offered less frequently to older patients, although numerous studies demonstrate good functional outcomes and improved quality of life even for patients over age eighty.[23] As less-invasive treatments such as angioplasty and stenting become more common, we can expect these treatments to become standard care and be offered to all, even the very old. Improvements are also likely in pharmacological approaches to preventing clots and plaque. Gene transfer might be used to reverse atherosclerosis inside a blood vessel or replace scarred heart tissue with functional cardiac muscle. But preventing atherosclerosis is still the most effective approach, and drugs have been shown to be very effective in reducing "bad" cholesterol (LDL). For those with diabetes, good management of the disease is essential to preventing the complication of diabetic vascular disease, which can also cause heart attacks.

STROKE

Preventing stroke is an important medical goal in treating patients with high blood pressure. Effective hypertension management, often with multiple medications, requires close monitoring. One recent advance involves administering thrombolytic (clot-dissolving) drugs during the acute phase of a stroke. Dissolving clots that obstruct blood flow to the brain can minimize or prevent damage to brain tissues. This treatment involves a risk of brain hemorrhage, so an immediate CAT or MRI scan of the brain is recommended. To reduce disability and death from strokes, the public needs to learn to react to signs of a possible stroke in the same way that we have been taught to react to a possible heart attack. In the future, stem-cell therapies may allow the replacement of brain cells damaged by stroke.

VISUAL AND HEARING DISORDERS

Vision and hearing disorders cause a significant loss of function in the elderly and unfortunately are commonly accepted as among the inevitable consequences of aging. For vision disorders, cataract surgery and laser treatment are quite successful; these are the most common procedures paid for by Medicare. Diagnosis and treatment of glaucoma, another major cause of blindness, is more difficult.[24] Because visual loss from glaucoma can halted but not reversed, early detection is important.

Advances in the study of macular degeneration, the leading cause of blindness for those over age sixty-five, are likely to have an effect over the next few decades.[25] Recent reports of in-vitro gene transfers are one promising development.[26]

Cochlear transplantation is a promising surgical technique for elders with hearing loss. Commonly used for younger patients, this surgery has proved highly successful in older adults as well, with significant gains in independence and quality of life.[27] Bioengineering approaches to hearing loss are also on the horizon.

Medical professionals and insurance systems (including Medicare) do not consider these disorders to be as serious as other medical problems. Traditional Medicare will cover surgical procedures related to vision but will not cover enhancement devices like glasses or hearing aids. However, these sensory functions are essential to maintaining independence as well as mental and social functioning that can reduce the risk of depression, a serious psychiatric disorder common in old age.

WHY MEDICATIONS MATTER

Prescription drugs are in the forefront of recent advances and promising developments in medicine. They are at the core of several treatments and make possible new interventions that were formerly beyond the physician's abilities. Drug research and development is monumentally expensive but in the long run can save lives, distress, and money by eliminating the need for invasive procedures and hospitalization. Observing the integration of pharmacology into nearly every aspect of medical therapy, especially for those over sixty-five, shows the sense and imperative for calling on Medicare to support a comprehensive and cost-effective way to help pay for prescription drugs. The two most important means of achieving this—negotiated price discounts and selective coverage of the most cost-effective medications—have both been ruled off-limits in the 2003 Medicare Modernization Act because of pressures from drug companies.

But simply adding a prescription drug benefit is not enough to modernize Medicare. Many of the medical advances outlined above require primary care, careful follow-up, and continuous monitoring. Team-based care management for chronic conditions, rehabilitation, and prevention should be the mainstream in modern geriatric medical practice. Expanding coverage to promote these aspects of care is just as important as pharmaceutical or surgical interventions. To ensure that all older citizens have access to the scientific advances that are at the heart of modern medicine,

Medicare needs to acknowledge modern geriatric principles and shift its coverage priorities accordingly. Expertise in geriatric medicine, combined with flexibility in covered benefits, is essential to a modern version of Medicare.

What Scientific Progress Means for Medicare

This quick overview of some of the frontiers of modern geriatric medicine shows scientists conducting cutting-edge research to understand, prevent, control, and cure age-related diseases. Whether these developments truly lead to more successful aging will depend on whether Medicare makes treatments available. Most important, none of these disorders occurs alone; all are best managed with comprehensive, coordinated care that prevents complications and enhances function. Traditional Medicare is designed to pay for episodic treatments and not comprehensive management, as I discuss in chapter 4.

Healthy aging does not come free. In the end, progress depends on cost and on who will pay. Is this a social goal that warrants spreading the cost over the whole population equally? Or should those who can pay be in the vanguard of those who benefit? We can expect the costs of care to grow, potentially without limit, until we decide as a society that we can no longer afford it. With health-care spending already accounting for more than one-eighth of the U.S. economy and growing, there is increasing discussion about rationing care to control costs.[28] Rationing appears unjustifiable when there are abundant opportunities to economize by improving efficiency and effectiveness in the health-care system, especially by care management and careful, evidence-based prescribing. Our new longevity suggests that we should reconsider our priorities before deciding where to set limits. There is less reason now than ever to impose rationing by age-based criteria. On the contrary, considering the many possibilities for substantial benefit, we might approve a growing share of Medicare in the overall health-care budget, especially if we knew we were getting value and quality for the money we spend.

CHAPTER 3

Ensuring Quality of Care for Elderly Patients

Although the United States spends far more on health care than any other nation, citizens generally cannot expect a reliable quality of care. Experts agree that fundamental changes are needed in the organization and delivery of health care, but they do not agree on what changes are most likely to lead to the desired improvements. Health professionals are challenged to bring the benefits of effective health care to the public while avoiding unnecessary and harmful interventions, medical errors, and preventable complications.

Because of the complexity and chronic nature of their illnesses, people covered by Medicare are more susceptible to gaps and problems in quality of care than any other age group. At the same time, they possess a unique advantage: they are beneficiaries of the country's only program of universal health care, a system powerful enough to support real and positive change.

The principles of geriatric medicine provide a firm foundation for defining quality care for an aging population and reflect concerns common to all patients. Geriatric medicine emphasizes care that is patient-centered: patients are entitled to care that is customized to their needs; continuous, coordinated, and cooperative attention from practitioners; and timely access to information so that they can control the care they receive.

A Framework for Quality Care

The Institute of Medicine (IOM), in its 2001 report *Crossing the Quality Chasm,* provides a framework for an ideal health-care system, focusing on four major challenges that threaten the quality of care.[1]

I. GROWING COMPLEXITY

In the past two decades, geriatric medicine has evolved from a specialty that concentrated on reducing the use of futile interventions at the end of life to a field with an armamentarium of new medications and technologies that help people live longer and healthier lives. Research and technology promise quality treatments that were previously unthinkable. The very success of this ongoing transformation in medicine raises the first point of concern.

The training and efforts of individual practitioners are more intense than ever, but no physician can possibly keep up with the volume of clinically relevant scientific information that arrives in a variety of publications every day. Physicians need the tools of information technology and an interdisciplinary team to help them process and use this information in the clinical setting.

Addressing the growing diversity of specialties and resulting fragmentation in medical care is a problem not fully addressed in current practice. Specialization reduces the burden of expectations on any one practitioner, but all efforts ultimately center on the individual patient. Manual paper records and the culture of individual decision making by physicians are no longer adequate in an environment demanding rapid information access, interactive diagnostic systems, and a team strategy. With advances in our understanding of the basis of disease and treatment and in the development of technologically complex therapies, more specialists and specialized equipment will be involved: no one will know everything, not even in his or her own area of expertise. Leadership by a primary-care physician who has geriatric expertise will become more important than ever to ensure quality health care for the elderly.

Developing an integrated system of care is critical for meeting the multiple needs of an aging population. Electronic information systems are beginning to play a vital role. Grants from the John A. Hartford Foundation, beginning in 1991, assisted the development of "community health management information systems" in several states.[2] Such systems allow more efficient coordination of care and also provide data on quality, costs, and use of services that can be used to guide quality improvement and purchasing. There is a pressing need to go further, however, and develop a national health-information infrastructure that allows interactive clinical decision making and transferable electronic medical records. Although elements of such a system are developing, particularly with computerized physician order entry (CPOE) and adverse drug event (ADE) alert systems for prescribing medications,[3] the current patchwork of multiple, incompatible systems will eventually prove a liability. Government investment in and coordination of system standards is necessary and is already under way in Canada, Australia, and the United Kingdom.[4]

Moving toward an electronic medical record (EMR) for patients is a common item on the agenda of current health-care reformers. As a patient consults with various providers, fragmented records hinder the coordination of care and increase the probability of preventable errors. As we age, our medical histories become more complex, yet patients cannot be sure that every encounter with a doctor, nurse, social worker, or pharmacist will refer to the same medical record. Time-consuming repetition of information is burdensome in itself and risks omissions due to lapses of memory, selective interest, or simple recording errors. Among the advantages of EMRs are features such as electronic checklists and interactive alerts that help the physician gather all relevant information.[5] Transmitting medication orders electronically allows for checks on accuracy, dosage, allergies, and potential interactions with other drugs the patient is taking.

Health-care professionals have been working toward a transferable EMR since the 1970s. Sophisticated EMR capabilities are standard at Mayo Clinics across the country. Other developed models exist at the Veterans Health Administration (VHA, also known as the VA) and the Department of Defense (DoD).[6] The VHA system allows patients to look up their own medical records. The DoD is currently expanding from regional systems to a universal system with lifelong patient records. In 1997 Kaiser Permanente completed development of an EMR with embedded decision-support tools for its Pacific Northwest facilities.[7] Kaiser, a large not-for-profit health system, is now spending $2.5 billion to convert its entire system, encompassing more than eight million people, to EMR.[8]

Less comprehensive efforts, many not much more than paper-and-pencil methods transferred to the computer with simple word-processing or database programs, are also being developed.[9] Numerous software companies offer EMR packages, especially since the full implementation of the federal Health Insurance Portability and Accountability Act (HIPAA) in 2002. Because all providers who bill Medicare or Medicaid are now required to process claims electronically, electronic data systems are nearly universal for billing purposes, if nothing else. Unfortunately, as an unfunded mandate without national coordination, HIPAA has generated an enormous variety of electronic systems. Although certain customized EMRs can prove useful in promoting efficiency and quality for the isolated clinician,[10] the kind of transferable EMR that can truly help to integrate care delivery remains rare.

Our fragmented, competitive health-care system offers no built-in incentives for investing in coordinated electronic systems. A sophisticated EMR is beyond the financial means of most medical practices, even larger clinics and hospitals. Moreover, the self-contained systems of Mayo, Kaiser, the VHA, the DoD, and others are incompatible. Sharing information among nursing homes, ambulance personnel, home-care organizations, and other community-care facilities, relying primarily upon oral and paper communication, remains fraught with the risk of errors. Until standards are established for an electronic information resource that can be used throughout the health-care system, any organization that invests in a singular product must worry about becoming obsolete, like a railroad with the wrong gauge track.[11]

2. INCREASE IN CHRONIC CONDITIONS

Medical advances in acute care have led to a new awareness of chronic conditions. Earlier, when more people died suddenly of heart attacks in their forties or fifties, they were spared exposure to serious chronic conditions. As people live longer, nonfatal but disabling chronic conditions linked biologically to the process of aging, such as arthritis, Alzheimer's disease, Parkinson's disease, depression, and diabetes, have become more common. Improved management of these conditions has allowed people to live with them longer.

In addition, advances in diagnosis and medical treatment mean that other serious illnesses can be controlled before they become life-threatening; thus a new array of chronic conditions has emerged. Cancer, for example, is often successfully treated; and while some people are completely cured, others live for years and even decades with a recurring cancer kept at bay by a combination of surgery, radiation, and chemotherapy. With close monitoring, early identification, and prompt treatment, individuals with cancer can go on with their lives for considerable periods. Similarly, heart disease, though still the nation's major killer, can be effectively treated and controlled. Treatments like heart surgery, angioplasty, medication, and changes in lifestyle allow people to live for decades with chronic cardiovascular disease.

These powerful developments in medical effectiveness led the IOM to name care coordination as a top priority for quality improvement.[12]

Nearly half the population—about 125 million people—lives with some type of chronic condition. About half that number live with multiple chronic conditions. Of the Medicare population, 88 percent are estimated to be living with one or more chronic conditions and 65 percent with multiple chronic conditions.[13]

Living with chronic conditions requires coordination of care over time and among multiple health-care providers. Yet physicians are not trained adequately in coordination, nor are health-care systems generally organized to accommodate it.

Diabetes is a good example of a chronic condition for which care coordination can drastically reduce the number of complications, including expensive hospitalizations. Programs involving regular outreach to patients, information systems, decision support for physicians and nurses, reminder systems for checkups, and interdisciplinary teams have shown better outcomes: lower blood sugar, lower blood pressure and cholesterol levels, better kidney function, fewer visual complications, and less vascular disease. The demonstrated effectiveness of coordination in this area reflects the concept of "prospective" or "anticipatory" care to prevent complications that might result in extra doctor visits or hospital stays. At present, however, most delivery systems and payment structures—including traditional Medicare—are based on an acute-care model that pays for responding to problems, not creating solutions. The doctor is paid only if a patient makes an office visit; the hospital is paid only if a patient is hospitalized.

Capitation—paying a set amount in advance to cover all necessary medical care—attempts to reverse the wait-and-see incentive. (The term *capitation* is often used interchangeably with *prepayment*.) Under capitation, providers profit by keeping the patient healthy. Unfortunately, there is concern that many health maintenance organizations (HMOs) have used capitation to reduce rather than coordinate care, a perception that has led to a backlash of patient-protection legislation and a retreat from capitation as a viable payment method. Health-care experts are now intent on finding a "functional equivalent"[14] to capitation that encourages conscientious care management and pays for the time involved in keeping patients healthy, maintaining function, and relieving suffering.

The increase in chronic conditions in the population demands a form of health-care organization and payment that fosters communication and outreach. For many chronic illnesses like diabetes, heart failure, or Alzheimer's disease, careful communication with the patient and family can improve health and reduce the need for office visits and hospital admissions, thereby reducing overall health-care costs.

3. POORLY ORGANIZED DELIVERY SYSTEMS

Health-care delivery in the United States is highly decentralized. One-fourth of all physicians still practice alone, and another one-fourth practice in groups of fewer than ten. If physicians in federal employment and institutional settings are excluded, nearly 80 percent practice in groups of fewer than ten.[15] As a consequence, most physicians in the community do not have the information technology or the interdisciplinary teams necessary for effective care coordination.

Technologically advanced in particular treatments and devices, the health-care system remains organizationally backward. Many patients and their families feel the health-care system is a nightmare to navigate. They find it impersonal; they do not have access to their own records; important information has to be endlessly repeated and is often forgotten, lost, distorted, transcribed incorrectly, or left behind when the setting of care changes. Transferring from the hospital to a nursing home, for example, produces a fresh record, extensive new forms, and selected information from the patient's previous history. In most systems, gaps and confusion in care occur during a transfer because no one has responsibility for ensuring the transfer of all the appropriate records.

Edward Wagner, who has spent his career studying the management of chronic illnesses, identifies five elements required to improve outcomes for the chronically ill:

Evidence-based practice. Explicitly incorporate evidence-based, planned care into practice through guidelines and protocols based on research.

Teamwork. Organize practices to meet the needs of patients who require more attention, incorporating a broad spectrum of staff skills, flexibility in the use of resources, and closer follow-up. Multidisciplinary expertise is usually essential, with careful coordination and communication among team members.

Patient empowerment. Communication with patients should give systematic attention to the patient's need for information to help manage behavioral change for disease prevention or to cope with disabilities.

Clinical integration. To benefit from advances in science and technology, patients must be able to see the right specialist at the right time. Their needs can be accommodated with large, integrated systems in which many specialists work together, or by Internet computer support. Physicians and patients together should have access to objective information that allows them to identify specialists with the best outcomes of care.

Electronic medical records. Supportive information systems can help to track patients who need various kinds of prevention reminders and follow-up care. Similarly, electronic transfer of medical records can reduce redundancy in forms and laboratory tests and avoid the loss of important clinical information.[16]

Wagner's goals for chronic care are consistent with the principles of modern geriatric medicine and the aims of IOM's *Crossing the Quality Chasm.* Endorsement of the same principles by different groups testifies to the wide range of consensus among medical and health-care policy experts. The vision of where we want to go is relatively clear.

The current problem is that highly organized systems are not rewarded. Instead, strong financial incentives exist to overutilize expensive technology in discrete episodes of acute care, viewing the patient as a case of the moment rather than an individual with diverse and continuing needs, interests, and personal accountability for health. Meeting the challenge for quality health care will require systemwide change. Medicare could provide the leadership for the rest of the health-care system if it could overcome political obstacles while maintaining its universal and equitable population coverage.

4. LACK OF INFORMATION TECHNOLOGY

Modern information technology already stands out as a resource central to the delivery of quality health care. Information technology improves the efficiency of claims processing and other administrative tasks and facilitates data collection and quality assessment. The signal advantage of information technology in health care—of critical importance for safety and quality—occurs in the clinical setting. The transferable electronic medical record improves the quality of patient information and access across multiple settings. Moreover, embedded decision tools clearly improve the quality of treatment decisions.[17] Physicians and patients together may review options, acquire up-to-date evidence of recommended treatments, and, through an interactive computer system, ensure that all appropriate details have been considered.

These capacities can be especially useful for patients with multiple chronic conditions who receive care from different specialists and other providers. Of foremost importance is the ability to monitor a patient's drug regimen, which tends to become increasingly complex and problematic as a patient ages. A computerized order entry system can monitor drug combinations and assess the potential for adverse reactions before they occur. Unfilled prescriptions can be checked to be sure that a patient is on track with a vital treatment. For example, the physician can monitor whether the patient is refilling prescriptions on schedule and so can be assumed to be taking the medication correctly.[18]

Training will be required to incorporate information technology into clinical practice patterns, especially with respect to communication with patients and colleagues. Information tools will facilitate the use of evidence-based practice in clinical decision making, but management to ensure physician support is essential, and teamwork is required to support the system.[19] Corollary functions might be added to improve long-term supervision of health for the individual patient, tracking trends in the community or analysis of rare conditions. Collating data from individual records would allow closer attention to general quality measures and costs. The possibilities are vast, and, even with a standardized system, customized options are bound to proliferate.

For patients with computer access, information systems can extend the clinical relationship, allowing twenty-four-hour access to the patient's own medical record and, for example, rapid and convenient access to lab results. Under the Health Information and Portability and Accountability Act, patients' access to their own records is now mandatory in any case. Making computers available to patients in the office will be a necessary part of the system, along with providing access to physicians, nurses, pharmacists, and others. Tailoring the patient record for patient access requires another set of decisions to enhance comprehension and avoid undue anxiety.[20] Advisory information and specific protocols could be included in the record to promote care management at home. E-mail enhances the ability to ask and answer questions in a more relaxed way, without the time pressure or anxiety people often feel when on the telephone or in the exam room.

From the patient perspective, of course, the use of information technology raises a major concern about privacy. The confidentiality of personal health information is a fundamental value of medical ethics. Inappropriate disclosure of medical information can have serious consequences, such as social stigma, employment discrimination, and the loss of health insurance. Federal rules implemented as a consequence of HIPAA have changed the way health information is managed, with an emphasis on patient privacy. The most significant effect is the clamp put on the transfer of patient records from one provider to another, requiring the often impossible condition that the patient appear in person to sign a release. New developments may allow the use of electronic signatures for patients to signify approval from a remote location, and encryption of electronic records may ease concerns over confidentiality. The extensive changes mandated by the new rules have led to confusion, but refining standard procedures should gradually result in a system that works.

The compelling advantages of electronic information systems for health care make it difficult to understand or accept the extreme backwardness that prevails. Although most health-care organizations have some kind of website, few personalize information access for patient use; and almost none have automated service functions such as physician orders, medical management, and medical records. Health care lags behind most other industries in its use of information technology. In 1996, health care organizations spent an average of $500 per worker on information technology compared with, for example, $12,000 per worker spent by financial investment and security systems. In a 1999 survey of investment in electronic systems by the U.S. Department of Commerce, health care ranked thirty-eighth in a field of fifty-three industries.[21]

The largest obstacle to the application of information technology is cost. However, neglecting technology also incurs significant costs, which are becoming increasingly apparent. Improvements in health-care quality as well as cost control will be thwarted as long as substantial investment in information technology is delayed. We are attempting to operate a complex system without the proper tools.

Quality Goals in Geriatric Medicine

Outside the clinical setting, information technology is being used to collect and disseminate data about the quality of care. Idealized views of consumer choice often envision a prospective patient shopping for providers on the Internet, comparing cost and quality. A large proportion of baby boomers are certainly comfortable with computers, but even the most discerning health-care consumer faces enormous difficulties in this endeavor.

First, we know little about the types of information patients will care about and how much data can be posted before it becomes simply overwhelming to the average person. About half of those with Internet access do look up health information, and half of those claim that the materials have affected their decisions about treatment and care; but this is not to say they have been able to judge the quality of the information or of health-care providers. For Medicare, improved educational materials have had a moderate effect,[22] but, as the former Centers for Medicare and Medicaid Services (CMS) administrator, Thomas Scully, complained, "There is definitely a problem when 65,000 seniors a day are calling for information about Medicare."[23] Rather than simplify the system and absolve beneficiaries from so many important choices, his proposed solution was to pepper the media, bulletin boards, and mailboxes with yet more information. We still don't know how patients really use extensive data about provider quality.

Providing information to individuals in the belief they will become prudent purchasers and force quality improvement by their informed selection—as if they were picking out a household appliance—is unrealistic. Even with recent cutbacks, Medicare allows a wide choice of physicians (unless one is enrolled in a managed Medicare HMO plan). But how can the prospective patient determine quality in a way relevant to his or her immediate needs? How can individual physicians be compared with multispecialty groups? Advocates of consumer choice claim that exposing the individual to an increasing share of the costs will encourage discrimination and careful purchasing, but does it? Health care is much less susceptible to detached choice and objective indicators than other purchases, and it is more likely to be influenced by subjective factors, such as personal recommendations, trust, loyalty, and fear. Moreover, such decisions have long-term implications. Mistaken choices in health care may not be remedied as easily as choosing a different restaurant after a disappointing meal.

Third, according to an IOM report of studies appearing in the *Journal of the American Medical Association,* nearly half of the adult population in the United States is barely literate: 21 percent (40 to 44 million people) are functionally illiterate, and another 25 percent (50 million people) are marginally literate, unable to synthesize information from technically complex or lengthy texts.[24] This 46 percent is reported as functionally illiterate with respect to health care, relying upon oral instructions and faulty recall (hence the volume of telephone calls by beneficiaries to CMS). This half of the population is not going to be online making critical decisions.

Certainly, electronic systems may improve access to information for patients, but this should not be understood as the primary goal (which is, rather, coordination of information to improve quality), as suggested by market-oriented theorists intent on fixing market failure in health care by empowering consumers. Medical information is complex, and most individuals are neither equipped nor inclined to act as prudent purchasers. Businesses that purchase insurance on behalf of their employees do have the ability to use quality data, and in some cases they have become influential in pressing health systems and physicians to meet stated criteria for quality measurement and clinical outcomes. Medicare can similarly be seen as a powerful purchaser exercising leverage on behalf of its beneficiaries: there are attempts now by Medicare to require certain quality measures and even to pay more to providers for better performance.

When health-care outcomes data is used to select care providers, the process is called *measurement for selection*. Such selection processes by purchasers are powerful tools in the quest for quality improvement, but it is not clear who should be regarded as the prudent purchaser. Even for Medicare, with the government at the apex of the system, the locus of authority over purchasing decisions is not easily located. Since 1997, Medicare has required HMO contractors to provide quality indicators from the standard Health Plan Employer Data and Information Set (HEDIS), which is supposed to allow consumers to compare alternative plans. The HEDIS measures are also supposed to be used by the HMOs to evaluate their network of providers. Yet this approach does not seem to be working any better than end-consumer choice. Alliances between HMOs and hospitals are determined mostly by cost and location rather than by quality.[25] The organizations that collect and use information on quality of care are the health plans, and they operate under pressure from government regulations and the expectations of employer purchasers. HMO contracts with providers stipulate that they must provide appropriate data for measuring quality, submit to utilization review, and institute quality-improvement programs. Likewise, providers who accept Medicare patients must submit to cooperative arrangements with Medicare's contracted Quality Improvement Organizations (QIOs) in each state.

Performance information captured by quality indicators, such as HEDIS measures, display such data as rates of mammograms and flu shots administered, complications among diabetes and heart patients, surgical infections, and mortality rates. HEDIS has expanded over the years, and in February 2003 eleven new measures were introduced, including two treatments for children, management of osteoporosis and urinary incontinence for older adults, chemical dependency services, and three measures of customer service.

When these data are collected and fed back to providers for internal review and comparison with other providers, the process is called *measurement for improvement*. This procedure is based on models of continuous quality improvement that have been proved effective in many other industries, from services to manufacturing, and is beginning to be more widely accepted in health care. Results from many sources show that providing this kind of reliable information about performance does lead to improvement. Organized problem-solving teams involving hospital or clinic administrators enhance the process.

Publicized report cards that actually rank local providers (usually hospitals) are a popular way to present quality measures. Media attention, both local and national, is usually part of the process: *Consumer Reports* and *U.S. News and World Report* are familiar sources. The ranking in the report cards is typically easier for the public to understand. Publication of the reports may also motivate the lower performers among the providers to improve quality by the mere fact of public scrutiny.[26]

However, the report-card strategy often creates a negative environment that sometimes leads to providers' refusing to treat difficult patients who might make outcomes look worse. Conflict also frequently arises over the legitimacy of the quality measures. The result does not necessarily improve quality if there is no economic advantage to investing in the effort.[27] In the confusing health-care marketplace, ambiguity as to the purpose of the report card increases the potential for negative responses. Who is the real consumer? Why publish data on quality that are difficult to interpret and may be misleading when selection processes by employer groups, just like those of HMOs, ultimately refer to cost and ignore quality indicators anyway?

Even without an adequate system in place to use quality indicators in purchasing decisions, a great number of health-care quality initiatives and legislative mandates are being churned out. We need to stop and ask how these can be useful without a clear idea of who will use the information and why. Such information is expensive to produce, particularly in health care, where assessing outcomes is neither straightforward nor always amenable to quantification. In some cases, doubts are raised whether a quality indicator actually correlates to a measurable patient outcome at all. Perhaps, once again, the prominent orientation toward market theory is leading policy makers to believe that this expensive information will function as an invisible hand, creating market competition on the basis of quality. When will that be? Closer analysis suggests that a definite purpose, identifiable players, and organizational capacity are necessary to make information perform any function at all.[28]

Regulatory forces and professional values may continue the quest for quality even in the absence of effective market forces. Quality indicators are already being provided to satisfy accreditation bodies and government regulations. With the National Committee for Quality Assurance (NCQA) accrediting health plans, and board certification for physicians increasingly linked to quality-of-care measures and quality improvement strategies, the culture of health care has probably reached a point beyond which pressure for quality measurement will continue even if it is not linked to financial rewards. Still, that link could strengthen the forces of accountability.

THE RELATIONSHIP BETWEEN QUALITY AND QUANTITY

The IOM report suggests that a large part of the problem of quality of care in the United States is the amount of ineffective or potentially harmful care that is provided. With health-care spending predicted to increase to 17 percent of the gross domestic product by 2011, it becomes ever more critical that each health-care dollar is used to provide quality care.

Health-services researchers have observed broad regional variations in health-care spending patterns across the United States. For example, in 1996 Medicare spending in the Miami region averaged $8,414 per enrollee, compared with an average of $3,341 per enrollee in the Minneapolis region.[29] These differences do not seem to be due to differences in the price of services or in levels of illness or socioeconomic status. Instead, researchers point to differences in the overall quantity of health services provided and to the greater proportion of physicians and medical subspecialists in higher-cost areas. Savings of as much as 30 percent of Medicare spending might be possible without sacrificing quality and might also lower the incidence of unnecessary intervention.

A recent study examined the relationship between health-care spending and health outcomes for Medicare recipients in different regions.[30] Researchers looked at variations in end-of-life spending for Medicare patients hospitalized with hip fracture, colorectal cancer, and acute myocardial infarction. Outcome measurements included the type and frequency of services received, quality of care, and access to care. The study found that patients in higher-spending regions received about 60 percent more care, in the form of more frequent physician visits, more tests, more minor procedures, and increased use of specialists and hospitals. However, quality of care was no better, and there were no differences in access to care in the different regions. Furthermore, there was no relationship between spending and five-year mortality rates, functional status, or patient satisfaction.

In applying these findings to Medicare policy, it will be necessary to convince patients that more care is not necessarily better care. It is possible to deliver high-quality services and produce excellent outcomes by doing less but doing it right.[31]

DEFINING QUALITY

In *Crossing the Quality Chasm,* the IOM challenged the health-care system to continue to reduce the burden of illness, injury, and disability and to improve the health and functioning of the nation's citizens. Concerns for quality in health care involve a vast array of specific treatments and practices. To help direct the many activities for quality improvement in all areas, IOM formulated six broad aims as points of reference. The six aims assert that health care should be:

Safe—avoid injuries to patients from the care that is intended to help them.

Effective—provide services based on scientific knowledge to all who would benefit, and refrain from using services that do not work.

Patient-centered—provide care that is respectful and responsive to the individual patient's preferences, needs, and values.

Timely—reduce waits and harmful delays for those who receive and give care.

Efficient—avoid waste and duplicative or unnecessary interventions.

Equitable—provide care that does not vary in quality because of gender, ethnicity, geographic location, or socioeconomic status.

These aims reflect undisputable values. Everyone wants health care that meets these goals. Yet we are clearly not getting it. Research and personal testimony from Medicare patients confirm there is a long way to go to reach any of these goals in a reliable manner. Medicare is the one example of a health-care system in the United States potentially capable of decisive and uniform effort to achieve whatever ends it might approve; yet, even here, a sense of fragmentation and disorientation persists.

Much of the literature about improving quality of care actually reflects the principles of good geriatric medicine. In this sense, the concerns of the Medicare population reflect basic concerns for primary care and quality care applicable to everyone. Geriatric medicine asks for care based on (1) continuous healing relationships; (2) customized services devoted to individual patient needs, which also allow the patient to exercise control over care; (3) access to information that is accurate and timely and shared with patients and families; (4) interdisciplinary teams and coordination of services across different settings; (5) anticipation of needs to avoid complications and exacerbations of chronic illnesses; and (6) cooperation, communication, and collaboration among specialists working toward patient-centered goals.[32]

These principles are consistent with the IOM aims for quality care and with Wagner's components of good chronic care. Such consensus provides a strong basis for public agreement that Medicare should be structured to meet them; it should also make older people, their families, and health care providers profoundly dissatisfied with the chaotic and fragmented care most Medicare patients experience.

Medicare is built on traditional, physician-centered practice and a reactive model of acute care. Both of these elements impede the goals of good geriatric medicine. Ideas for reforming Medicare to better meet the needs of its beneficiaries are quickly saturated with a flood of details, and it will be useful in the ensuing chapters to maintain a vision of the clear targets presented here. These are the standards that will help chart our course.

CHAPTER 4

Care Management

The Key to Modern Geriatric Medicine

Quality health care is difficult to judge in the abstract. Statistics help to quantify the overall situation and alert us to problem areas, but the desire to improve and the motivation to provide the best health care possible comes from the stories of people like you and me. Stories give care management a face that moves us and can identify areas where we should be concerned. Consider the following case.[1]

Mrs. Clay is an elderly widow who lives alone in substandard housing. She has seen a cardiologist and a urologist but has no primary-care provider. Following an increasing number of falls and the onset of major depression, she was found by a neighbor three days after a fall. She was brought to an emergency room with serious dehydration and a hip fracture. After a three-month hospital stay, partly in intensive care, Mrs. Clay was stable enough to be discharged to a nursing home.

Medicare paid for the first sixty days of Mrs. Clay's hospitalization, less a deductible of about $800. For the following thirty days, her hospital stay cost her about $200 per day. Medicare covered an initial period of rehabilitation at the nursing home. However, when it appeared that Mrs. Clay was not improving, Medicare discontinued payment: the program will not pay for skilled nursing care for patients who "plateau" or whose stay exceeds one hundred days. Because Mrs. Clay has no financial reserves, her nursing-home stay was paid for by Medicaid.

Mrs. Clay's experience included other complications, including two emergency hospital visits for pneumonia during her time at the nursing home. While older people are at risk for pneumonia, physical activity and good hygiene reduce that risk, and early attention by a geriatrician could have prevented the need for Mrs. Clay to go to the emergency room. Much harm and expense could have been avoided through greater attention to her functional decline and better coordination of her medical, housing, and social-service needs. Economic disadvantage and social isolation—common among elderly women in the United States—likely exacerbated her condition.

All older adults, regardless of economic resources, are vulnerable to similar health problems and treatment issues. Primary and community-based care should focus on maintaining function and anticipating common problems. Flexibility of medical coverage is essential to allow early intervention. Physicians should be reimbursed for monitoring and communicating with the patient at home and working with nurses, social workers, and other caregivers to manage frailty and prevent complications and unnecessary hospitalizations. Ideally, a primary-care provider trained in geriatrics would have monitored Mrs. Clay's condition and ensured that she received attention that could have prevented or reduced the severity of her health problems, including physical therapy after her injury; treatment for depression; evaluation of her home for fall hazards and for ways to accommodate her physical limitations; assessment of her drug regimen; and the provision of an electronic alert device or buddy system to ensure a prompt response to an emergency.

Unfortunately, Medicare does nothing to encourage proactive attention to progressive impairments. Both in the original mandate for Medicare and in today's modified version, the fee-for-service arrangement provides treatment only when the patient gets sick or injured and arrives at the clinic or emergency room. For Mrs. Clay, this solution was almost too late.

We know that something is wrong with a system that chooses to spend money on hospitalizations and nursing-home care rather than preventive interventions, personalized care management, and home health programs. We know we could do better at giving older adults the care they really need. How can Medicare change to accomplish the goals of modern geriatric medicine? How can we produce the coordinated care older people need? And how can the nation ensure that older citizens will be able to afford it?

Two Scenarios of Care Management

Tilda Anderson was seventy-seven years old and moderately overweight when she was diagnosed with diabetes and high blood pressure. The conditions were identified during a regular visit with her internist. Mrs. Anderson received counseling from both her physician and a nurse specialist to help her understand how diet, physical activity, and body weight affect her medical conditions. She signed up for peer support, nutrition classes, and exercise instruction and was able to lose ten pounds and start an exercise regimen. Her blood pressure dropped to normal, but her blood sugar remained slightly elevated. She was started on a mild oral medication to control her diabetes and scheduled for regular monitoring of her blood sugar, including home monitoring, which allowed her to keep it within the desired range. She received reminders for vision checks and foot care, since the small blood-vessel damage that comes with diabetes often leads to visual problems, kidney failure, and circulatory problems affecting the extremities.

Mrs. Anderson was under a good deal of stress because her husband, who was ten years her senior, had chronic congestive heart failure. He was cared for by a visiting nurse who monitored his weight and vital signs and adjusted his medications. He stayed in touch with his physician—a specialist in cardiology—through e-mail reminders, telephone interactions, and scheduled office visits. In the past year, however, Mr. Anderson had become increasingly forgetful; he was likely in the early stages of Alzheimer's disease. He woke up frequently at night, interrupting his wife's sleep, and she worried that he would leave the house and get lost. She was not sure whether to sleep in a separate bed so that she could get some rest or stay with him to monitor his movements.

The cardiologist consulted with the geriatrician, who is part of the prepaid, integrated, multispecialty health-care system, and arranged for a day hospital to provide respite care for Mr. Anderson several days a week. This allowed Mrs. Anderson time to rest, take care of herself, and visit her family. Tired out by the exercise activities and interaction at the day hospital, Mr. Anderson was more likely to sleep through the night. He received new medications that ameliorated some of the symptoms related to his stage of Alzheimer's disease. Because bringing him to the doctor's office took an extraordinary amount of planning and energy, the medications were administered and monitored for potential side effects by a visiting nurse.

As Mr. Anderson's Alzheimer's disease progressed, the health-care system's palliative care team cared for him at home until it was clear he needed to be admitted to a long-term care facility. The same doctors and nurses continued to care for him, providing relief for his shortness of breath and confusion. Mrs. Anderson was able to visit and provide emotional support. Eventually, he died peacefully, with his family gathered around him, according to the wishes expressed in the living will that he had written many years before.

After Mr. Anderson died, Mrs. Anderson's appetite declined, and she had difficulty sleeping. The nurse who called to follow up on a missed appointment thought she sounded confused and her words a little slurred on the phone. A visiting nurse found she had been drinking sherry and eating poorly. She had also stopped taking her diabetes medication, and her blood pressure was out of control. Mrs. Anderson received treatment from a psychiatrist, who prescribed an antidepressant medication that has few adverse side effects and helped her cope with this period of grieving. She also joined a support group of recently widowed women.

With social support and input from the people she has met through the widows' group, Mrs. Anderson decided, at age eighty, to move from her large house to an assisted-living retirement community nearby, so that she could stay close to her family but also have ready access to emergency care, meals, housekeeping services, and stimulating activities and social interactions. Her physician, nurses, and other members of her health-care team continued to care for her after this move. The assisted-living facility provided transportation to medical appointments, removing one of the barriers to keeping these appointments.

This story could have unfolded in a very different way. In fact, the following scenario is more likely in the United States. Mrs. Anderson was alerted to her serious health problems, but the Andersons struggled to pay for the medications they needed. Mr. Anderson's congestive heart failure was managed by a well-trained doctor; but the multiple specialists did not communicate with one another and failed to anticipate problems, so Mr. Anderson often ended up in florid pulmonary edema, gasping for breath. Four to six times a year, an ambulance took him to the emergency room, where he was admitted to the hospital and treated.

Mrs. Anderson was given medication, and a couple of pamphlets about the importance of exercise and diet, and scheduled for a return visit. But she was unable to exercise or lose weight, especially with the hectic schedule and stress produced by Mr. Anderson's frequent visits to the emergency room. She put on more weight and needed increasingly heavy doses of medication. In order to afford her prescriptions, she began skimping on other things; but she also reduced her medication. Neither the diabetes nor the hypertension had obvious or immediate symptoms, and she reasoned that if she felt all right, then she could skip the occasional dose without a problem. One day she awakened unable to speak and paralyzed on one side. She was rushed to the emergency room, where it was discovered that she had had a stroke and her blood pressure was extremely high.

She recovered some of her function from the stroke but was ultimately unable to care for herself, much less for her sick husband, who was now also beginning to show signs of cognitive impairment. The only answer was for Mr. and Mrs. Anderson to sell their house and move to a nursing home. While there, Mrs. Anderson developed chronic renal disease because her diabetes had not been treated adequately. She had to go onto dialysis. Her vision failed because of diabetic complications, and she suffered from pain in her legs that led to vascular complications. One leg was amputated below the knee. Mr. Anderson's dementia worsened, and he was hospitalized more frequently for heart failure and pneumonia. Since he saw a different group of doctors each time, and his wife herself was disabled and incapable of speaking for him, he was intimidated and suffered, alone and confused, for a long time before he died.

This second version of the story is all too common in the United States. Not only is it tragic, but it is avoidable; and it is more costly than the care-management approach of the first scenario. Even with enriched services and care coordination, preventive care is much less expensive than the multiple hospitalizations needed to deal with acute-care crises. Medicare, as other insurance, is only a payment mechanism, but how we pay for care sets up clear incentives for how doctors and hospitals organize the care. Medicare needs to change, and our health-care system with it, to provide higher-quality care that is patient-centered and based on the principles of geriatric medicine.

Modern Geriatric Medicine

Modern geriatric medicine aims to improve or maintain functional status by maintaining continuity of care, preventing and managing chronic age-related conditions, and providing for dignity and relief of suffering at all stages of illness.[2] Physicians and their patients have only recently begun to realize that caring for older patients requires specific expertise. The concepts of geriatric medicine offer a set of established principles and tested strategies that should guide any discussion of the nature of insurance coverage for older citizens.

A new understanding of healthy aging has begun to reverse the traditional assumptions that associate old age with inevitable deterioration, illness, and disability. Home care and therapy services can help people continue to live full lives even with age-related conditions. Simple physical activity, for example, helps prevent the loss of physical condition that leads to serious decline, exacerbation of medical illness, and repeated hospitalizations. But preventive physical therapy is not considered medical treatment by Medicare and is therefore not covered. Medicare has not managed to keep up with advances in geriatric medicine and mostly gives providers financial incentives that emphasize acute hospital stays and treatment of short-term illnesses.

Traditional medicine and Medicare still fail to recognize that maintaining function is as important as treating specific diseases. Routine office visits and hospital stays present good opportunities for early detection of illness or functional decline. The most effective model involves collaboration among a multidisciplinary team of geriatricians, nurses, nurses' aides, social workers, physical therapists, and other health professionals. Geriatric assessment, a tool that provides information on a patient's general functioning, is important in planning care for elderly patients. Geriatricians look not only for treatable diseases but also for the syndromes that impair function, like frailty, confusion, urinary incontinence, postural instability, and falls. Assessment enables early intervention to prevent or delay more serious conditions.

Geriatric medicine is based on interdisciplinary coordination. Access to care and coordination and continuity of care among different settings, providers, and procedures requires extensive communication among team members, patients, and families. Care management may involve custodial home care, medications, psychosocial counseling, and the provision of devices to assist mobility, hearing, and vision. In contrast, episodic care involving multiple providers too often causes problems like harmful drug interactions or overmedication, which can lead to other forms of illness, such as depression and dementia.

Medicare is not structured to pay for interdisciplinary care management. Contact with the patient by telephone or e-mail, for example, is essential but not covered. Physician home care visits are reimbursed at a minimal rate, and physicians are not reimbursed for transportation time when they visit patients in nursing homes. Because of the obstacles to providing care in different settings, good physicians may place a patient in a hospital simply to maintain continuity of care, even when conditions might have been managed more effectively and economically in a nursing home or in the patient's own home.

Geriatric medicine relies heavily on nonmedical services provided by professionals such as social workers, nutritionists, and physical therapists.

Social workers, for example, help patients and families make treatment decisions and find and coordinate community services. Nutritionists and physical therapists help older adults maintain functional ability. These services are usually not covered by Medicare. We must recognize they are as integral to successful geriatric care as the strictly medical aspects of intervention are.

Older people need access to both advanced medical services and a system organized for interdisciplinary, comprehensive care management, which, ideally, includes electronic patient records and an ordering and tracking system for prescription drugs. Such infrastructure to support health care is still rare, existing only at government-run veterans and military hospitals, in larger integrated systems like the Mayo Clinic, Intermountain Health Systems, and Kaiser Permanente, and in a few other hospital systems.[3]

COORDINATING CARE

Quality of care has not been high on the agenda for Medicare reform. Policy makers are primarily concerned with controlling costs. The Medicare managed-care initiative implemented in the Balanced Budget Act (BBA) of 1997 was an effort to both improve quality and control costs. Managed-care organizations (MCOs) that take financial responsibility for Medicare enrollees have an incentive to improve health and reduce expensive treatments. Unfortunately, the ideal is not working as well as intended. Under the Medicare+Choice program (M+C), costs have risen, and quality has not improved.

M+C enrollment peaked at about 17 percent in 1999 and declined steadily to about 10 percent of the eligible Medicare population in 2004. During the program's first five years, MCOs have continually reduced benefits and canceled policies, creating a sense of uncertainty that threatens to reduce participation rates even further. Geographical variations in the availability and cost of Medicare MCO plans add an element of unpredictability and inequity.[4]

By restricting enrollment and offering competitive premiums, many MCOs have attracted healthier enrollees,[5] but they have found it necessary to restrict expenditures further by cutting back on extra benefits like drug coverage, which are important to beneficiaries with chronic illnesses. It remains to be seen whether the new Medicare Advantage private plans will fare any better. As in other markets, and particularly with health care, people want security and predictability.

For the Medicare population, special expertise in geriatric medicine and chronic disease management is essential. Some of the Medicare + Choice failures were probably due to lack of investment in this area. These MCOs may have been unprepared for managing the special needs of older adults and for providing resources and flexibility for appropriate care management. Too often MCOs control costs simply by restricting care; this is not care management. MCOs that are more concerned with their bottom lines than with the quality of their patients' lives have added to the mistrust many Americans feel toward managed care.

The revolution promised by managed care has, thus far, largely failed. Paying providers by capitation—a set amount per person per month— is no longer a preferred strategy. Negotiated fees and diagnosis-related group–type payments per episode are now the norm for the industry. The innovation shown in prepaid systems that manage an entire delivery system instead of just the insurance provides a more enduring lesson. Ensuring appropriate care can reduce unnecessary and more expensive treatments. In this context, there are good examples showing how managed care can really manage care and not just manage cost.

Models of case management, or care management, usually involve a nurse or social worker responsible for coordinating the patient's care. This extra attention helps to reduce unnecessary services, identifies gaps in care, and gives the patient an advocate for access to certain services. This commonsense model of managed care has been the subject of much research. Results are mixed. Some studies show improved outcomes, and some show reduced costs; others show neither. This kind of research is complex, and clear outcomes are hard to achieve, especially when function, quality of life, satisfaction, and peace of mind are taken into account—all harder to measure than quantitative changes in lab tests, mortality rates, and major cost reductions.[6]

PRIMARY CARE

Good primary care for older people (and indeed anyone with chronic conditions) and good geriatric medicine are essentially the same thing. Both require a single point of contact through which care can be coordinated. The lack of continuous primary care is one of the major deficiencies of the United States health-care system.[7] Such care is particularly important for elderly patients with multiple conditions that require a balance of sometimes competing treatments and medications. Primary-care physicians trained in geriatric medicine can provide Medicare beneficiaries with expert advice about their overall care management.[8] This might come as a relief to those older adults who travel from specialist to specialist with no single trusted doctor overseeing their care.

Patient-protection laws in some states have begun to ensure that physicians have the right to advocate care for patients and oppose restrictive rules by the MCO insurer. Restrictions on referrals to specialist care and diagnostic testing are also being loosened. Such patient protection, however, varies from state to state and from contract to contract.[9] And although these laws aim to promote the interests of patients, they may have unintended negative consequences. Many consumers don't realize, for example, that a wider choice of specialists means sacrificing the idea of carefully coordinated care within a unified system that shares medical records electronically and in which physicians from different specialties communicate with each other about each patient.

One challenge in treating older adults is maintaining the optimal care balance between the patient's primary physician (usually an internist, family physician, or geriatrician) and the numerous specialists seen for chronic conditions and other age-related illnesses. In some areas, such as cardiology, specialists may be more familiar with the latest research on how to treat specific chronic conditions and disabilities.[10] On the other hand, older people are likely to have several conditions needing specialist attention; moreover, most patients value the relationship with their primary physician and like to receive health care through one stable source. This potential conflict points to the importance of communication and teamwork in geriatric medicine. All members of a care team, including the primary physician, specialists, nurses, and social workers, must communicate with each other and with the patient to ensure that each member is satisfied with the patient's treatment plan. Traditional Medicare does not adequately reimburse for this kind of staff communication, even within a single hospital.

One way to incorporate care management into traditional Medicare is to pay for it separately. Additional case-management fees are already instituted in certain Medicaid programs, usually in rural areas.[11] Care providers are reimbursed separately for the time involved in arranging referrals to social service providers, and similar measures.

Several "care oversight" codes currently exist in the schedule of Medicare payments, but they are reserved for patients requiring home care or hospice services. They do not include routine outpatient care management and do not cover the costs of an interdisciplinary team that includes a nurse and social worker. People with chronic conditions, including most Medicare patients, would benefit substantially from this kind of extra attention. Improved reimbursement for care management would allow a physician to counsel patients more fully, which, in turn, would enhance self-management of conditions at home and the ability to recognize and treat problems early. Extra attention can reduce serious complications, improve conditions for long-term nursing home residents, and allow more complete preventive measures.

Models of Coordinated Care

Good models of care management for older adults exist and should serve as instructive models for Medicare. For instance, the nonprofit sector supports stable group- and staff-model prepaid systems (where doctors are paid by salary, and patients pay a monthly fee instead of fee-for-service) that have been extraordinarily successful in providing well-coordinated care. Equipped with complete information about the status of their patients and the quality of outcomes, care providers can cooperate to provide seamless, personal care to each patient. To coordinate care in this way requires some restriction in the choice of participating providers. Within a large group, however, patients can choose from a number of physicians. These systems provide cost-effective, high-quality, multidisciplinary care management across the continuum of care, integrating preventive, acute, and long-term care.

U.S. citizens have been led by unfortunate stories of "bad" managed care to believe that having a choice of as many physicians as possible is the way to get the best quality medical care, yet the evidence indicates quite the opposite. The broad networks of physicians that are the most prevalent model cannot hold their physicians accountable for the quality of their performance, the level of their skills, or the ways in which they manage chronic illness. Consumers have very little information about the quality of individual providers and even less about the ability to coordinate care.

In contrast, an HMO or multispecialty group practice, like the Henry Ford system based in Michigan or the Kaiser Permanente system in several states, has a defined panel of its own providers (approximately 1,200 physicians in Henry Ford and 12,000 in Kaiser Permanente). These systems can maintain an intensive quality-improvement process that gives physicians reliable and rigorous feedback about their performance. Integrated health systems also support the development of coordinated interdisciplinary teams, which can be ideal care models for people with chronic and complex illness.

Unfortunately, these integrated models have been written off by many in the policy world as obsolete. Nothing could be farther from the truth. They are the only organizations that can really deliver on the promise of affordable, modern medical care for older Americans. The American health-care system will benefit by using these models as benchmarks in designing a Medicare for a positive aging society.

DEMONSTRATION PROJECTS

In 2001, Medicare awarded contracts for fifteen coordinated-care demonstration projects. These experimental contracts, mandated by BBA 1997, were divided into two categories: disease management for major diseases (mostly congestive heart failure) and case management for multiple chronic conditions. The law also called for a preliminary study of best practices in coordinated care to help direct the demonstrations. The study provided a comprehensive illustration of familiar points in successful care management.[12]

Disease management focuses on individual diseases and emphasizes commercial companies that interact with patients separately from the physician. The Medicare Modernization Act of 2003 mandates a huge investment in this strategy. Since many older people deal with more than one chronic condition, however, these programs are likely to have limited effectiveness. They do not support the integration of multiple providers into a coordinated care system. This is the difference between care management (a principle of modern geriatric medicine) and disease management (a strategy to reduce Medicare expenses).

A recent study of coordinated care includes two observations underscoring the need for care management: "Many, if not most, persons with chronic illness receive neither high-quality care nor care that meets their needs"; and "a small proportion of chronically ill persons incur the large majority of health care costs, and . . . many unplanned hospitalizations of chronically ill persons appear to be preventable."[13] Successful programs generally involve a team of practitioners or a number of individual providers in active communication and coordinated by a case manager or primary care physician.

The study found that the setting and reimbursement system of the programs made a difference. The capitated organizations, like HMOs, had an incentive to screen new enrollees and actively identify high-risk individuals who could most benefit from care management; whereas hospital-based programs and those operating under fee-for-service arrangements identified participants from among elderly patients already entered in the system or from referrals.

Taking care of older adults, especially those with chronic conditions, requires a proactive model of health care. Studies indicate that older adults with chronic conditions are most likely to follow treatment plans if they receive regular follow-up care, whether from their physician or someone with less clinical training. Follow-up mechanisms do not need to be face-to-face visits. Telephone calls or e-mails can be effective. Regular contact serves several purposes: not only does it allow the provider to monitor symptoms and medication, but it also reinforces the patient's self-management, which is a critical component in the treatment of chronic conditions. Since traditional Medicare does not reimburse providers for contact that is not face-to-face, it does not encourage optimal management of chronic conditions. Instead, it gives physicians a financial incentive to wait until a patient calls with a crisis and treat acute symptoms as they arise.

One innovation to facilitate communication involves group meetings. The Group Health Cooperative in Seattle, Washington, established mini-clinics for frail elders and people with diabetes. Patients with similar health needs meet for group meetings with a team of practitioners that supplement individual appointments. Kaiser Permanente in Colorado established a similar model with a Cooperative Health Care Clinic (CHCC), where seniors with at least one chronic condition and relatively high levels of health care use meet monthly in groups of fifteen to twenty with a team of practitioners. Early data show that CHCC patients were more satisfied, more active in their self-management, and used some health services less than a comparison group. These management programs for chronic conditions are examples of follow-up and teamwork in modern geriatric medicine.

INTEGRATING LONG-TERM CARE

Long-term care includes the services of family caregivers, paid home-health aides, nursing homes, and other subacute facilities helping people to perform basic daily activities. Such assistance is largely ignored by Medicare. In 1965, long-term care was considered an essentially non-medical service. Today, long-term care is one of the most important forms of care for older adults. Long-term care is also expensive, placing the kind of catastrophic burden on families that Medicare was supposed to alleviate.

In 1999, approximately one-fifth of the population aged sixty-five and over required assistance in at least one activity of daily living (ADL) or lived in an institution.[14] ADLs include such essential daily activities as eating, bathing, and going to the toilet. Of those with at least one ADL limitation, about half have been found to have substantial long-term care needs.[15] An additional portion of the population needs help with instrumental activities of daily living (IADLs), tasks related to independent living, including preparing meals, managing money, shopping, performing housework, and using the telephone.

Improved medical care could help many older persons maintain their independence, but the overall challenge of caring for those who need assistance will increase as the proportion of the population over age eighty-five continues to grow. Attention to this issue is bound to intensify as the baby boomers age. However, the national commitment to chronic care, as represented in nursing-home and home-health expenditures, is falling behind expenditures in other sectors of health care. A definite commitment to chronic care has yet to emerge.

Considering the major role of Medicaid and state programs in the existing provision of long-term care, there is some debate over whether the national government should expand its role in this area and supplant the states' authority.[16] Leaving aside the current severe crises in state finances and the natural limits on the scope of commitment possible at local levels, the argument for Medicare's managing long-term care hinges on the interface between acute and chronic conditions. The coordinated-care demonstration projects implemented by Congress show a growing awareness of such efforts in controlling costs, but adequate care management is not really possible without a commitment to supporting long-term care.

INTEGRATING COMMUNITY-BASED CARE: PACE

One example of a successful care-management project is the Program of All-Inclusive Care for the Elderly (PACE). Funded by both Medicaid and Medicare, PACE is designed to delay or prevent the necessity of placing older adults in nursing homes. Day health centers provide a comprehensive range of preventive, primary, acute, and long-term care services in addition to group activities, recreation, and meals. Multidisciplinary teams of practitioners include physicians, nurses, social workers, and physical and recreational therapists. Door-to-door transportation for participants is provided. CMS currently reports twenty-five approved PACE sites, each with about two hundred members.[17]

The program provides capitated payments from which all costs must be met, including acute care and hospitalization. Enrollees must be eligible for nursing-home placement according to state Medicaid criteria. The program assures all services covered by Medicare and Medicaid but is free to provide any additional innovative services it determines to be valuable for the health and independence of its enrollees.

BBA 1997 changed PACE from a demonstration project to a permanent program under Medicare. States were granted the option of offering PACE to their Medicaid enrollees. Although the law now allows the model to be freely adopted, expansion has been slow. Apparently, no one on the financing end is making a profit that makes it worth replicating on a larger scale.

The average PACE enrollee is eighty years old, has eight medical conditions, and needs help with three ADLs.[18] Despite their frailty, enrollees have shown lower hospital and nursing home use and higher satisfaction than people who applied to PACE but later decided not to enroll.[19]

An example helps make the point. An eighty-five-year-old woman with moderately advanced Alzheimer's disease is being cared for at home by her husband, who is mentally intact but has severe osteoarthritis and moderately severe congestive heart failure, which make it hard for him to get around or do any heavy work. He assures their principal physician and nurse that he and his wife both have living wills and do not want to end up "dying in a hospital attached to a bunch of tubes." He hopes that he will not be forced to place his wife in a nursing home but worries that his medical problems may prevent him from caring for her.

If the wife were placed in a PACE program, the couple would receive services that would help the husband take care of her at home. For instance, she would receive help at home with bathing. Assistance with household chores and meal preparation would relieve the burden on the husband. Transportation to a day center for a day or two each week or month would allow the caregiving team to monitor the couple's chronic conditions and medication (both would join the program). The excursions would also give the couple an opportunity to engage in social activities and participate in group counseling.

Because the couple have indicated in their living wills that they wish to avoid intensive-care hospitalization, the PACE program will not be obligated to pay for this expensive service when either of them becomes critically ill and likely to die. Otherwise, the PACE physician and team are expected to use high-cost services when appropriate. The diversified team structure allows providers to try other options first. An episode of pneumonia, for example, could be treated in the home with intravenous antibiotics, oxygen, nursing, and physician services.

Traditional Medicare will not pay for any of the home-care services or day-care activities that would support this couple and help them continue to live together at home. Under traditional Medicare, if the wife developed an infection and needed treatment, her husband would be obliged to call 911 to have her brought to the hospital, where she would probably be admitted and treated with intravenous antibiotics. A confused Alzheimer's patient in the hospital can be a nightmare for both patient and staff. Keeping an intravenous line secure can require restraints, which may frighten the patient enough to necessitate sedation. Sedation leads to inactivity and the possibility of bed sores and aspiration of fluid into the lungs, which would complicate the pneumonia. Dementia and confusion are also likely to increase in a strange environment. Medicare pays for such hospitalizations, but the cost, in both money and suffering, is likely to be greater than if the patient could be cared for at home.

In scenarios like this, PACE can help patients maintain a higher degree of control over their lives and their care and thus keep them in the community as long as possible. Saving money by restricting high-tech care can be successful, both morally and medically, if high-quality home and community-based care are provided. The only way to do this well is by investing in a structure that allows relationships to develop between a team of providers and patients with a similar range of needs. Group activities need to be combined with personalized attention, since the real needs of patients—especially those with chronic disease—are extremely varied.

PACE exemplifies the focus on team-based care most appropriate for geriatric medicine. The program also combines the idea of primary care coordination, utilization management, and, most important, a productive interface between acute and chronic care and a capacity to meet ADL needs, which remains particularly elusive in traditional health-care delivery. The question remains how the experimental design of PACE, or even Medicare + Choice, with its endeavor to manage care, may be used to shape traditional Medicare, in which most of the nation's forty million beneficiaries are still enrolled.

Managed care is probably essential to a Medicare program that works to provide modern geriatric medicine and sustain optimal quality of life as we age, but it must be done right. The prominent mistakes of commercial managed care that puts costs above care have conveyed the wrong message to much of the American public.

CHAPTER 5

Palliative Care

Many people on Medicare are confronted with serious and potentially lethal illnesses: an eighty-eight-year-old woman with dementia and congestive heart failure is hospitalized with pneumonia; a sixty-five-year-old man is diagnosed with inoperable brain cancer; and a seventy-year-old woman is diagnosed with leukemia and vows to fight her illness with all available medical technology. How each person faces his or her condition and chooses treatment strategies depends on that person's diagnosis, prognosis, personal values, and age. Some will choose the most aggressive, high-tech curative treatments available despite the risks and potential side effects. Others will embrace different goals, seeking to avoid suffering or the risk of dependency and foregoing potentially life-prolonging treatments. In some cases, as with the woman with dementia, the person may live for many more years, although she or he may no longer be capable of making such choices.

These widely varying cases above are all excellent candidates for palliative care, defined as the comprehensive management of a patient's physical, psychological, social, and spiritual needs. Although palliative care is commonly associated with treatment at the end of life, any person with a serious or life-threatening medical condition may benefit from its principles, which involve a patient-centered approach, pain and symptom control, family involvement, and compassion. Choosing palliative care does not mean that the patient gives up access to active medical treatment. In all cases, palliative care focuses on comfort and the relief of distressing physical and emotional symptoms. With today's medical technology, no one should suffer from medical conditions, including at the end of life.

Palliative care as a medical movement in the United States originated in the early 1970s, when Dame Cicely Saunders, the inspirational founder of St. Christopher's Hospice in Britain, gave a lecture at Yale University about caring for dying patients. Her talk stimulated the Yale community to start a hospice program. The first hospice, a facility devoted to providing palliative rather than aggressive curative treatment, was established in Connecticut in 1974.

The more recent history of the palliative-care movement has been driven largely by Medicare funding. In 1978, the Health Care Financing Administration (HCFA) funded twenty-three selected hospice programs and evaluated their cost-effectiveness in a national study. Medicare began to cover hospice care in 1983. The hospice benefit may be chosen when life-prolonging measures have been exhausted. Patients who qualify receive a full range of medical and social services, including outpatient prescription drugs, home health services, physician and skilled-nursing services, pastoral care, and counseling, and their survivors receive bereavement services.

In 1997, the Robert Wood Johnson Foundation funded the Last Acts project, designed to educate the public, policy makers, and health-care professionals on issues surrounding end-of-life care. The Last Acts Palliative Care Task Force developed the following precepts of palliative care:

· Respect patient goals, preferences, and choices

· Provide comprehensive caring

· Utilize the strengths of interdisciplinary resources

· Acknowledge and address caregiver concerns

· Build systems and mechanisms of support

These precepts should be practiced throughout the scope of any serious illness. Palliative care is life-affirming and regards dying as a natural process that is a profoundly personal experience for the dying person and his or her family.

Although pain relief is important, the goals of palliative care reach far beyond pain management. For people with serious illnesses, symptoms such as breathlessness, nausea, sleeplessness, confusion, and depression can be as distressing and as prevalent as pain. These conditions should also be treated with consideration and expertise. The intensity and range of palliative interventions may change as an illness progresses. The complexity of care may increase. Eventually, the focus shifts to the process of dying with emphasis on achieving a death that is consistent with the patient's values and expressed desires.

Trends in Palliative Care

Why do we need a public movement to help us learn how to die? The idea seems preposterous until we realize that people today die differently from our forebears: because we live longer, we tend to die older, of different causes, and in different environments. In 1900, people often died at home, surrounded by their families. Physicians routinely comforted the dying at the bedside. Over the past century, medical and public health advances have almost doubled the average life expectancy, from less than fifty years to nearly eighty.[1] People who die when they are old are likely to experience a long period of functional decline before death and thus require intensive personal care and well-coordinated medical care. As medical advances have allowed us to delay death, we have moved it from the home into institutions. Although most people say they would prefer to die at home, mortality data for 1999 show that among those aged sixty-five and over, only 21 percent of deaths occurred at a residence; 41 percent occurred in the hospital, another 28 percent at a nursing home, and 7 percent in an emergency room or clinic or on the way there.[2]

Our increased longevity has also changed the social and financial needs of the dying. As more people live to a very old age, they are more likely to live alone, without relatives nearby. If a frail older person lives with a spouse, that person is also likely to be frail and incapable of providing full-time care. It is no wonder we need to relearn how to care for the dying. Because we are dying a new kind of death, we need different end-of-life measures. Providing well-coordinated care, including home care, has become a new challenge. We need to learn how to help people manage comfortably and retain reasonable functionality and quality of life before death.

MEDICARE'S HOSPICE DESIGN

Medicare rules make hospice care available to patients whose physicians certify they have a life expectancy of six months or less, who agree to receive only palliative care, and who have a full-time primary caregiver.

In 1983, the Medicare hospice benefit dramatically redefined hospice care in the United States. Because the Medicare benefit emphasizes home care, hospices that had initially been built around an inpatient model needed to change the way they operated to qualify for reimbursement. In 2000, hospices cared for an estimated seven hundred thousand patients, with 96 percent receiving routine home care and 56 percent dying at home.[3]

Nearly 25 percent of Medicare beneficiaries who died in 2000 received hospice care, compared to 9 percent in 1992.[4] Admissions to hospice care more than tripled in that period, and the service gradually changed from one catering primarily to terminal cancer patients to one accommodating a fairly even balance of patients with cancerous and noncancerous diagnoses, including heart disease (10 percent), dementia (6 percent), end-stage kidney disease (3 percent), and end-stage liver disease (2 percent).

The Medicare hospice program works well for people with fairly predictable diseases, especially end-stage cancer, but because it is intended for people who will die within six months, and because it strictly limits inpatient or technical care, it is less helpful for people with diseases that are not as predictable, like heart disease, or those with a long period of decline, like Alzheimer's. To avoid being charged with Medicare fraud, providers may hesitate to encourage patients to enter hospice care until death is clearly imminent. As the percentage of noncancerous diagnoses among hospice patients has risen, the average length of service has declined, from sixty-four days in 1992 to forty-eight days in 2000. Those dying within two weeks of admission—predicted by a diagnosis of congestive heart failure, myocardial infarction, or lung cancer—rose from 21 percent in 1992 to 30 percent in 2000.

With many diseases, it is impossible for physicians to feel confident predicting death within six months. Although more people now benefit from hospice services through Medicare, the six-month rule has led to a drastically short period of care in spite of a "clarification" by CMS (then HCFA) in 2000 that the rule refers only to the probability and does not absolutely preclude longer periods of service. Reluctance by some providers to refer a patient to hospice care may be due to a reluctance to be seen as "giving up." Consequently, many patients simply receive no hospice care or are delayed until their final days, when opportunities to reach spiritual and emotional closure and benefit from palliative care have been diminished.

A good illustration of these points recently appeared in the literature, indicating the difficulty and anguish imposed by basing treatment decisions on the estimated time to death rather than the condition of the patient:

Our mother was an 87-year-old Alzheimer's patient as she approached the final month of her life. During her final month, mother was hospitalized for about 2 weeks before dying of pneumonia and hypercapnia (respiratory failure). Generally, the care she received was good, as doctors, nurses, and technicians tried to keep her comfortable while attempting to keep her alive by balancing the levels of oxygen and carbon dioxide in her lungs. But toward the end, we became frustrated with attempts to keep her alive at the cost of increasing levels of pain. Two weeks before our mother died, we asked the attending physician in the hospital if it was time for hospice care, and she believed it was not. She said that in mother's current condition, most patients lived from six months to as long as two years. Had hospice care been started at that point, mother could have died peacefully and without challenges to the advance directive by medical personnel.[5]

Similar delays are caused by the Medicare requirement not to use any life-prolonging efforts, which neither physicians nor families are comfortable with. Some moderate life-prolonging measures, such as administering intravenous antibiotics for infections, can buy precious time for patients and families. These decisions need to be governed by the physicians and family who know the patient and the situation. Medicare eligibility rules rigidly limit hospice care to a certain type of dying patient, favoring those with a home, a family caregiver, or the means to hire a full-time caregiver, because it only pays for a few hours a day of professional care. Like many program eligibility criteria, the Medicare hospice rules have had unintended consequences, curtailing broader access to palliative care.

The hospice programs financed by Medicare are a good step toward public acknowledgment that people die and that care for the dying is a valuable aspect of health care. Hospice care now needs to be expanded to benefit more people. Further, we need to apply precepts of palliative care to all care, not just to care at the end of life.

Pain Management

Clinicians are making great strides in accomplishing the goals of palliative care. A few inspirational stories of successful programs have been collected in *Pioneer Programs in Palliative Care: Nine Case Studies* (2000), published by the Milbank Memorial Fund and the Robert Wood Johnson Foundation. Earlier, the Institute of Medicine provided a useful contribution with *Approaching Death: Improving Care at the End of Life*

(1997), which addresses quality, personal experiences, and models for organization, financing, and professional education. The second edition of the *Oxford Textbook of Palliative Medicine* (1998) provides a wealth of perspectives valuable for medical and professional education, including an international perspective and recognition of the collaboration required in a team of caregivers, including volunteers.

Part of the mission to improve quality and accountability in palliative care involves expanding the definition. Until very recently, palliative-care programs emphasized treatment of pain, but not in conjunction with attempts to cure disease. Beginning in 2001, the Joint Commission on Accreditation of Healthcare Organizations (JCAHO)—the organization that accredits most medical facilities in the United States—started assessing pain-management programs as part of its accreditation process. JCAHO's acknowledgment that pain management has an essential role in all medical facilities is an important step toward incorporating palliative care into mainstream medicine. We must hope that many of the hospitals and nursing homes now developing pain-management programs in response to the new standards will go further and develop programs that incorporate a full range of palliative-care services. Certainly the new standards will help focus attention on and underscore clinicians' obligations to patients.[6]

The Annual Survey of Hospitals by the American Hospital Association began tracking palliative-care programs in 2002 (showing data for 2000). At that time, 42 percent of U.S. hospitals reported a formal pain-management program (mostly consisting of educating staff); 23 percent offered formal hospice services, provided in the hospital or at home; and 14 percent offered a palliative-care program.[7] The 2003 survey (reporting data for 2001) showed 806 hospitals offering palliative-care programs, up from 668 the previous year.[8] An independent hospital survey by the Center to Advance Palliative Care, based at the Mount Sinai School of Medicine in New York City, showed that less than half of hospitals with a palliative-care or pain-management program provide consultation service to allow experts to assist in patient care across a spectrum of other specialties, less than one-fourth have dedicated inpatient units, one-third have community hospice services offered by outside contractors, and one-third have outpatient palliative-care clinics.[9]

Thus, although there have been some welcome developments, too few patients receive adequate end-of-life palliative care. In the early 1990s, the four-year Study to Understand Prognoses and Preferences for Outcomes and Risks of Treatments (SUPPORT) began an effort in teaching hospitals to document the type of care preferred by dying patients, compared to what they received.[10] Published results in 1995 showed that patients' wishes were frequently not followed, and pain was common. Half the patients able to communicate in the last three days of life said they were in severe pain. The study convincingly demonstrated the need for hospitals and health systems to pursue a higher standard for end-of-life care.

SUPPORT results helped educate physicians on the importance of good end-of-life care and the general inadequacy of this care. Many physicians became motivated to improve the end-of-life care they provide and have begun to do so. Such efforts may carry the medical profession to a higher standard for palliative care throughout the life span.

Models for Palliative Care

Most Americans say they would prefer to die at home. Nonetheless, depending on geographic region, 20 to 50 percent of deaths occur in the hospital, according to the *Dartmouth Atlas of Health Care 1999*.[11] The Dartmouth research shows a dramatic variation in the treatment of similar patients, even if populations are matched by age, demographics, and burden of illness. There is a positive relationship between the number of hospitals in an area and the likelihood of being hospitalized, including for end-of-life care. Absent other options, the hospital becomes the conventional place for certain kinds of care that might be provided more effectively outside the hospital. Similarly, the presence of too many specialists can affect treatment in ways that are neither cost-effective nor beneficial to patients.

The *Atlas* also shows the following.

· Among Medicare enrollees, 15 percent to more than 50 percent will experience at least one stay in an intensive-care unit during the last six months of life.

· Up to 30 percent of all Medicare enrollees are likely to be admitted to intensive care during terminal hospitalization.

· On average, 11 percent of Medicare enrollees will spend seven or more days in intensive care during the last six months of life.

When should death occur in the hospital setting? The answer depends on factors such as family support, the availability of community-based resources, patterns of illness, and financial resources. In any case, clinicians must be expected to provide good palliative care in every setting, whether at home or in a hospice, hospital, or nursing home. The following situations illustrate why people on Medicare need positive, realistic end-of-life options outside the home.

TERMINAL CANCER: NURSING HOME

Mrs. Porter is an eighty-eight-year-old widow dying of colon cancer. Her grown children live in other states. Although they call frequently, they cannot visit for extended periods of time. Mrs. Porter might find a hospital or nursing home a more supportive environment than her home. Even if she could afford a full-time paid caregiver at home, she would probably have fewer different types of social and caregiving contacts at home than in a structured caregiving setting. Unfortunately, most nursing homes are not equipped to provide the intensive, sophisticated palliative care that a terminal cancer patient requires. Because of cost and the Medicare restrictions, inpatient palliative care or hospice serves only patients with a short life expectancy (a few days to a week). If Mrs. Porter stays in the hospital, the cost will be exorbitant. If she goes to a nursing home, where staffing is inadequate to provide the care she needs, she is more likely to die alone and in pain. Under the current system, no good options exist for her.

TERMINAL CANCER: HOSPITAL

Mrs. Matthews is a sixty-five-year-old woman with late-stage ovarian cancer that has not responded to chemotherapy. Her physicians have told her there is no more they can do for her except keep her comfortable. She is eligible for hospice care, and the comfort care appeals to her. However, her seventy-year-old husband cannot care for her physical needs, and she feels uncomfortable having her children see her bloated body and care for her draining wounds. Instead, she chooses to enter a hospital-based palliative care program to allow professionals to care for her physical needs so that her family will have the time and energy to provide emotional support. The problem with this option is that if her life expectancy is greater than one to two weeks, hospital care will be unaffordable.

MULTIPLE CHRONIC CONDITIONS: NURSING HOME

Mr. Stein was a ninety-year-old widower with numerous age-related chronic conditions, including high blood pressure, Parkinson's disease, severe arthritis, and osteoporosis. He was also taking medication for depression. Two years earlier, he was hospitalized for pneumonia, which was treated with antibiotics. After he recovered, he was weak and required physical therapy in addition to close medical monitoring of his other conditions. Although Mr. Stein would have preferred to go home, he and his physicians determined that he would receive better care in a nursing home, since he lived alone and Medicare would not pay for a twenty-four-hour home health aide. As Mr. Stein's functional ability continued to decline, it became clear that he would not be able to return home. When he began to experience organ failure and became eligible for the Medicare hospice benefit, hospice professionals attended him in the nursing home where he eventually died. Mr. Stein was able to benefit from palliative care throughout his nursing-home stay. He was fortunate that the physicians and nurses at his nursing home were trained in palliative medicine and understood the importance of relieving distress, and that the hospice program was able to add to the nursing home's capacity to provide more intensive comfort care when needed.

ACHIEVING FLEXIBILITY

In the three cases above, only one patient was well served. Typically, nursing-home residents are undertreated for pain. Fewer than 5 percent of those dying in nursing homes are enrolled in a Medicare hospice program.[12] New JCAHO pain standards, though optional for nursing homes, may motivate more institutions to improve the way they diagnose and treat pain.

To accommodate the diverse needs of people with serious illnesses, pioneer clinicians are creating new models for the delivery of palliative care. Traditional hospice care, as defined by Medicare, needs to add the flexibility to pay for other options so that palliative care can be readily obtained in a variety of settings, including the hospital, nursing home, and the patient's home. The five innovative models of palliative care listed below are becoming increasingly common.

Consultation service. A team composed of physicians and nurses, typically with a social worker and/or bereavement counselor, sees patients who need palliative care anywhere in the hospital.

Dedicated inpatient unit. Beds for palliative care are clustered in one area of the hospital. A dedicated unit may be combined with the consultation service. A dedicated unit provides visibility and may enhance acknowledgement by hospital staff of palliative care as an essential service.

Combined hospice–palliative care unit. An inpatient unit serves both hospice patients and hospital patients with palliative care needs.

Community hospice–hospital contract. Through a contractual arrangement with a community hospice program, a hospital provides pain management, comfort care, and skilled terminal care in an inpatient unit. This model expands Medicare payment options available to hospitals for these palliative care services, as they are reimbursed (albeit inadequately) through the Medicare hospice benefit.

Hospital outpatient palliative care clinic. A clinic operates in conjunction with a consultative service or inpatient unit to provide continuity of care after discharge from the hospital. This model promotes care continuity and is often linked to physician and nurse home-visiting programs.

Special Needs of Older Adults

In many ways, geriatrics and palliative care are natural allies. Both areas of medicine emphasize the importance of continued function, comfort, and quality of life regardless of life expectancy. A geriatrician, for example, might recommend that an otherwise healthy eighty-five-year-old woman with severe arthritis consider hip or knee replacement surgery. Some might argue she is too old for major surgery or that arthritis pain is something old people need to live with; but a geriatrician is likely to advocate surgery if the patient wants continued mobility, as a successful outcome is likely, given providers with geriatric experience and expertise. Similarly, a physician trained in palliative medicine will try to make a patient as comfortable as possible in her last months, weeks, days, or even hours, when other physicians might already have insisted that no more can be done.

Palliative care and geriatrics also share the principles of flexibility: tailoring care to each patient's individual needs, treating multiple conditions, emphasizing communication between the physician and the patient and family, and relying on an interdisciplinary approach to care. With this in mind, principles of modern geriatric medicine can and should be incorporated into the palliative care of older adults.

In some ways geriatric medicine and palliative care define success differently. Geriatricians are trained to keep seeking ways to improve a patient's quality of life, whereas palliative medicine teaches the provider when to stop pushing. Among the hardest decisions a physician and patient can make together is when to stop seeking new interventions and accept the imminence of death. Palliative care requires them to confront and accept mortality and the limits of medicine. Facing this decision has not been part of the training of care providers in the last half-century.

Palliative care is sometimes withheld because of the implication that it means giving up. Certainly clinical choices in critical situations can be extremely difficult.[13] Aggressive treatment often involves uncertain outcomes and clashing opinions. A cascade of unexpected complications may irreversibly change the patient's condition. Uncertainty in a stressful situation often prevents the medical team from being able to define that turning point when palliative care, and death with choice and dignity, is the better option.

In other cases, there may be a bias towards undertreatment for those who are older or are cognitively impaired. Some studies have shown that very old people are undertreated for pain more often than younger patients. In one study of daily pain management for people with cancer in nursing homes, one-fourth of those aged sixty-five or over who reported daily pain were given no pain medication at all, not even Tylenol.[14] Older residents received less pain medication than younger patients and were less likely than younger residents to receive even acetaminophen as well as more powerful medication like weak opiates or morphine. Other studies also indicate that an estimated 45 to 80 percent of nursing-home residents experience significant levels of untreated pain.[15]

Pain management relies heavily on self-reporting of pain, and patients with cognitive impairment (generally associated with the very old) may be unable to communicate their levels of pain effectively. In a study of eighty-eight patients with recent hip fractures, all were undertreated for pain; but nurses gave patients with cognitive impairment less medication than patients without cognitive impairment, despite the fact that physicians had prescribed the same amount of medication for both groups.[16] Many other studies confirm undertreatment of pain for older adults.

A recent Harris survey found that one in five Americans on Medicare take analgesic medications several times a week. Two-thirds of those people had taken prescription pain medications for more than six months. Untreated pain can lead to serious complications and functional decline. Some consequences of chronic pain include depression, reduced social activities, sleep disturbance, and decreased mobility. Such problems may lead to more serious problems. When older adults are unable to exercise, for example, their muscles become weaker, leading to further risks associated with immobility, such as falls.

Although people of all ages can benefit from palliative care when they are close to death, older patients typically require a different model of care that mixes palliative care with life-prolonging measures. Consider the example of Mary Smelzer, an eighty-eight-year-old woman with congestive heart failure. Following a two-week hospital stay for pneumonia, her muscles are weak. Like many older adults, Mrs. Smelzer needs a combination of life-prolonging, preventive, rehabilitative, and palliative care. Life-prolonging measures include the treatment of her heart failure with oxygen and antibiotics; preventive measures include an annual mammography and flu vaccination; rehabilitative measures include physical therapy in her home to restore her mobility and daily functioning. At the same time, she is a good candidate for palliative care. She needs help from a social worker to write an advance directive and appoint a health-care proxy to make medical decisions for her if she becomes unable to do so. She probably needs treatment for depression, along with diuretics, oxygen, and low-dose opiates for her breathing difficulties. This combination of measures will improve her quality of life and sense of well-being and also reduce her dependence on others, but Mrs. Smelzer still needs help to carry on living at home. A home health aide could help manage her care and provide assistance with bathing and getting to the toilet, monitor her weight, and identify early signs of heart failure that would indicate a need to change medication.

Not all special needs are easily addressed by palliative care. Recognizing the appropriate moment to shift from acute treatment intervention to palliative measures is complex and not readily reduced to a protocol. We can recognize, however, that effort needs to be directed particularly to neglected and vulnerable populations. Greater emphasis needs to be given to a model of geriatric medicine that sees the older patient as a whole person with biological, functional, social, and spiritual needs.

Challenges for the Future

People in chronic pain use more health-care services than people without pain. By paying for medications and adequately reimbursing institutions and providers who deliver good palliative care, Medicare could help older adults to improve their quality of life and reduce their need for health services. Medicare needs to support adequate palliative care for all beneficiaries, not just those who are designated as terminal patients.

Care for the dying, in considerable measure, is publicly funded. Nearly three-quarters of those who die each year are over age sixty-five and on Medicare. Some are also insured by Medicaid or by programs for veterans or military personnel. The disenfranchised, who lack public or private insurance, may obtain health care at public safety-net hospitals. Government policies thus play a major role in determining the kind of care people receive at the end of life.

Medicare's hospice benefit has enabled more people to die with effective and compassionate care. Since Congress approved Medicare's hospice program in 1983, a palliative-care movement has gained momentum among physicians, nurses, patients, and friends and family members of the seriously ill, who recognize the need for high-quality palliative care. The good news is that the Medicare hospice benefit has provided a way to pay for good palliative care at the very end of life, especially for patients dying of cancer or AIDS, for which the course of illness is fairly predictable. The bad news is that the constraints imposed to limit costs have also limited access for a much larger group of patients who might benefit from these services and discouraged the interest of providers in developing the skills to provide palliative care.

By adopting some of the principles of the modern palliative-care movement and adequately funding a wide range of services, Medicare could exercise a profound influence on a new generation of caregivers and caregiving practices to relieve an unnecessarily large burden of suffering. To integrate palliative care into all areas of medicine, not just end-of-life care, however, reform must go beyond Medicare policies and reimbursement strategies. Other sources of leadership are also important. The education of physicians needs to change. There are currently too few training programs for palliative care at medical schools and training sites. Effective palliative care requires clinical skills and a knowledge of pharmacology, in addition to compassion and an understanding of medical ethics. Patients need to be educated, too, so that they can communicate clearly and demand relief from suffering. They should be given opportunities to plan ahead and obtain counseling to help them collaborate in defining care that is consistent with their values.

Current barriers to providing adequate palliative care in the United States include inadequate financing; a limited supply of trained physicians; few incentives for continuity of care; and cultural issues. Physicians, patients, and families often view death as a failure and are uncomfortable talking about it. The recommendations below summarize various strategies to improve Medicare policy and the professional environment for providing better palliative care.

Create a board-certified specialty in palliative medicine. This would focus attention on an existing knowledge base that is insufficiently understood, inadequately applied, and in need of growth. By acknowledging palliative care as a discipline, certification would support the credibility of palliative care with peers, patients, and families. Certification would also attract leaders to the field, nurture its development,[17] and define it as an area of expertise in the mainstream of medical practice.

Improve Medicare's physician payment system. Palliative-care providers are at a disadvantage under the Medicare physician fee schedule. Palliative care requires time-consuming consultations, often with both patient and family, which are reimbursed at rates considerably lower than procedural services that require similar investments of time. Medicare pays far more, for example, for a bronchoscopy and intubation leading to ventilator care in an ICU than for the discussions with patient, family, and consulting specialists that can avoid those intrusive, painful, and expensive preludes to dying.

Improve Medicare's hospital payment system. The current diagnosis-related group (DRG) system for Medicare hospital payments does not explicitly recognize the relief of suffering as a legitimate goal of hospitalization. That no DRG code exists for a patient requiring palliative care presents a significant barrier to providing end-of-life or palliative care. The idea of a payment code for palliative care raises a familiar objection: the concern that hospital staff would designate only some patients as "palliative" and not recognize that palliative care is an appropriate form of care for many others. (Prepaid or capitated systems allow flexibility because they aren't constrained by payment codes.) The challenge is the explicit acknowledgement of palliative care as a legitimate and necessary service. In the fee-for-service world, such steps begin to change the culture of care.

Relax Medicare's hospice eligibility rules. Currently, hospices fear they will be charged with Medicare fraud or abuse if they accept a patient to hospice who lives longer than six months after admission. In part as a result of this fear, too many patients enter hospice in the last days or weeks of their lives, long after they could have started to benefit from the team approach of hospice care. Hospice services need to be made accessible to people dying of any disease, including diseases less predictable than cancer. In addition, eliminating the requirement to forgo all life-prolonging services on entering hospice care could improve accessibility and relieve the anxiety for all concerned when coming to such a momentous decision. Eliminating the no-treatment rule would allow more flexibility and make the system more responsive to the real needs of patients and families.

Educate medical providers. Palliative care should be taught at the medical school and residency training levels. Good palliative care requires highly specialized knowledge of pharmacology and symptom management and cannot be learned in one or two lectures. Students and other trainees need to observe excellent palliative care given by interdisciplinary teams. Few teaching hospitals or residency programs currently have the kind of patient-care settings or faculty experts to conduct this kind of teaching.

Educate consumers. Patients and families are entitled to palliative care and the information they need to make difficult decisions. Health providers should be accountable for helping patients navigate the complex medical system and educating them to communicate effectively to obtain the best possible care. Quality-of-care measures by JCAHO or NCQA need to include evaluation of palliative and end-of-life care to motivate providers to pay attention to these services, and so that consumers can make informed choices.

Implementing these recommendations would make a reasonable start toward establishing a decent standard of palliative care. Today, with increased longevity and the aging of the baby boomers, we are at the brink of a new opportunity to create a society that is truly supportive of positive, productive aging—and dignified dying. The role of modern medicine in our increased life span and improved quality of life must also extend to a professional concern with reducing suffering.

CHAPTER 6

Medicare Coverage

Gaps, Limits, and Anomalies

If the principles of geriatric medicine are so straightforward, why does Medicare coverage not reflect this knowledge? Medicare coverage policies were developed in response to the prevailing health-care needs of the elderly nearly fifty years ago. Health services and needs have evolved considerably, but Medicare coverage has not kept pace with shifts toward prevention-oriented and chronic care. A brief look at the development and history of Medicare reveals the origins of this mismatch between traditional Medicare coverage and the best practices of geriatric medicine.

By the 1950s, medical treatment for everyone, not just the elderly, involved hospitals and their associated high costs. In 1958 an American Hospital Association (AHA) representative testified to the House Ways and Means Committee about the tendency "not only for persons to seek more hospital service, but for them to seek more complicated hospital services."[1] As more effective hospital treatments became available and patients and physicians began demanding them, costs became increasingly problematic for hospitals, which had generally provided free treatment to those who were unable to pay.

As a political maneuver, the supporters of the first Medicare bill lobbied for a limited hospital benefit. Theodore R. Marmor, a scholar of Medicare's history, writes that "the provision of 60 days of free hospital care only indirectly encourages preventive health measures and cannot allay financial problems of the long-term chronically ill. The hospital benefit was designed, however, not so much to cope with all the health problems of the elderly as to reduce their most onerous financial difficulties."[2]

Hospital bills were the most obvious choice for an initial benefit because they were the largest bills incurred during any spell of serious illness at the time. Also, because many of the medical advances at the time involved hospital-based treatments, the Medicare program promised to subsidize the continued advancement of hospital-based care by providing a stable funding source. The price of hospital care doubled between 1951 and 1961, partly because hospitals had more to offer: antibiotics for serious infections, new surgical procedures, and early versions of intensive cardiac care. All these treatments affected elderly people far more than others. Older citizens were hospitalized more than younger people. One in six older Americans entered a hospital in a given year, and they stayed in the hospital twice as long as those under age sixty-five.

An expanded range of effective hospital treatments increased public trust in professional medicine, and, with the 1946 Hill-Burton Act, federal promotion of hospital construction brought hospitals to the center of the health-care system. In 1959 an AMA representative testified to the House Ways and Means Committee: "There was a time when you almost had to drag the patient into the hospital. . . . Now it is rare you find anyone who wants to stay home."[3] This trend influenced Medicare's orientation toward acute care.

The original coverage guidelines established by Congress divided benefits into two categories: Part A provided hospital insurance (HI) and Part B supplementary medical insurance (SMI). Medicare Part A pays for a portion of inpatient hospital care and for a period of rehabilitation at a skilled nursing facility (SNF) after a three-day hospital stay, and for part-time home health-care and hospice care for those who meet certain eligibility criteria. Part A, similar to earlier versions of Blue Cross insurance in the private market, was designed to cover the catastrophically high cost of acute-care hospital stays. Part B, modeled on earlier versions of Blue Shield private insurance, generally covers 80 percent of physician services, both in the hospital and in the office or clinic. It also covers laboratory services in full and some home health-care and preventive services but does not pay for routine physical exams, outpatient medical or surgical services, or supplies (like prescription drugs), diagnostic tests, outpatient surgery, or some durable medical equipment, like wheelchairs and hospital beds.[4]

Enrollment in Part A is automatic at age sixty-five, so long as an individual (or spouse) has paid payroll deductions or self-employment taxes (FICA) for ten years. Part B, which pays for most outpatient services, is voluntary and charges a monthly premium. About 95 percent of the people on Medicare Part A are also enrolled in Part B. Anyone who chooses not to enroll in Part B when first eligible must pay higher premiums for later enrollment.

When first instituted, Medicare provoked an immediate rise in health-care use among the newly eligible older adult population.[5] Within six months, by June 1966, 17.6 out of 19 million eligible citizens had enrolled in Part B.[6] The number of enrolled beneficiaries has more than doubled since the program's creation, from 19.5 million in 1967 to 39 million in 2000, now constituting approximately 14 percent of the U.S. population. This increased enrollment is due in part to Medicare's expanding to include people with disabilities and end-stage renal disease (ESRD) and in part to greater life expectancy and demographic changes.

I use the term *traditional Medicare* to refer to the structure of the original program, established in 1965. Providers are reimbursed on a fee-for-service basis for delivering covered benefits that have been deemed "reasonable and necessary." *Capitation* and *prepayment* refer to the practice of paying a set amount per enrollee, in advance, to cover all needed care. Medicare Managed Care plans—such as Medicare+Choice (M+C) plans—are prepaid systems in which the plan contracts to provide a range of services that may exceed those covered by traditional Medicare. If these services cost less than the capitated amount, the plan makes a profit; if they cost more, the plan loses money. The advantage of prepayment is that the provider (a health plan or medical group) can decide what treatment the patient needs rather than leave it to Medicare to stipulate what is covered.

Coverage Gaps

Medicare payment policies affect medical decision making. Negotiated fees for designated services work fine so long as a person fits into the established categories. Too often, however, good geriatric medicine calls for care that falls outside the box defined by Medicare coverage. In general, an actuarial comparison to other health insurance plans shows that Medicare provides significantly fewer benefits than coverage for federal employees, small employers, or Medicaid.[7] The following story illustrates the possible consequences when a need for care arises.

MRS. PETERS'S COLLAPSE

Ellen Peters, an eighty-eight-year-old woman with moderate Alzheimer's disease, lives in her own assisted-living apartment. She receives frequent help from her three adult daughters, each of whom has medical problems of her own, as well as work and, for one, foster grandchildren to care for. After a minor fall, Mrs. Peters develops a vertebral crush fracture—a collapsed vertebra related to severe osteoporosis that sometimes occurs after a fall, or even after movements as minor as opening a window or turning to get out of bed.

Mrs. Peters is brought to the emergency room in extreme pain. The physician in the emergency room orders an X ray, diagnoses a vertebral crush fracture, and tells Mrs. Peters's daughter there is no reason to admit her mother to the hospital. The daughter is knowledgeable and assertive enough to insist on admission, knowing her mother cannot manage at home. The physician continues to argue that there is no reason to admit her because no treatment orders need to be written other than for pain medication and diet.

This physician clearly does not understand the principles of geriatric treatment. When he says her condition requires "no treatment," he means it requires no surgical intervention for which Medicare pays a defined fee. His lack of knowledge could have resulted in disaster for Mrs. Peters and her family.

A collapsed vertebra is extremely painful. The only cure is time. As she recuperates, Mrs. Peters will need frequent consultation with medical professionals to determine whether she needs different medications and physical therapy. She will need intensive and careful pain management, both for compassionate reasons and to prevent her from becoming immobilized. Without pain treatment, she would be unable even to get to the toilet, and with immobility her muscles would grow progressively weaker. She will also need to be carefully monitored for potential side effects of her pain medication as well as for possible adverse reactions with other medications she may be taking.

This example illustrates how Medicare has shaped the culture of medicine and health care in the U.S. Treatment is defined as anything Medicare pays for. Mrs. Peters's difficult situation would be considerably alleviated if she could obtain care for a week or two in a subacute rehabilitation unit. Such facilities are usually located in nursing homes. Nursing staff could help her keep up her muscle strength and monitor her pain treatment. By Medicare rules, however, rehabilitation services are paid for only if the individual is transferred to a nursing home from a hospital. Unless Mrs. Peters is first admitted to a hospital, her family will have to pay out of pocket or care for her themselves during her rehabilitation.

The policy requiring prior hospitalization for payment of subacute care is designed to prevent overuse. Rehabilitation and subacute services are helpful to maintain strength even for patients who do not have an acute illness, and payment for these services is viewed as a bad insurance risk without a definite adverse event, like a hospital admission, to justify it. But although the policy discourages overuse of rehabilitation, it induces overuse of hospitalization, since that becomes the only rational alternative for someone like Mrs. Peters, who does not really need hospital care but clearly needs close attention and physical therapy for a few weeks while she heals. Recognizing this absurdity, Medicare waivers are sometimes granted to organized health systems and HMOs to bypass the hospitalization rule and deliver patients directly from an emergency room to a nursing home. Relaxing the rule in this way saves money for the insurer while maintaining safeguards against overuse. Mrs. Peters, however, is not covered by a waiver: if she is not admitted to the hospital, she will get no rehabilitative care at all.

ADDRESSING CHRONIC CONDITIONS

Medicare coverage for acute-care costs has played an enormous role in alleviating the cost burdens associated with health care. Much of modern medical care, however, is provided outside the hospital. Complex, chronic conditions are often best treated through outpatient visits, medication, and close monitoring. Most illness in the elderly is chronic and therefore does not occur in discrete episodes with a clear beginning, middle, and end. Interactions with physicians are not always focused on making a specific diagnosis or performing a specific procedure or treatment but rather on managing symptoms, maintaining function, and preventing decline.

Medicare pays physicians and hospitals based on treatment episodes, like diagnosis and surgery for a benign tumor, repair of a broken hip, or treatment of an uncomplicated gall bladder infection. However, a patient with chronic illness, such as hypertension, coronary disease with heart failure, or osteoporosis, requires an ongoing relationship with at least one physician. Regular monitoring is needed in person, by phone, or even by e-mail to manage the patient's diet, activity and exercise regimens, and adherence to medication schedules, along with watching for drug side effects and interactions. Monitoring also involves reminders, moral support, and help in obtaining needed social services. These kinds of activities are not yet clearly part of the Medicare payment structure.

Medicare reforms have begun to address care management beyond the acute-episode model by acknowledging the value of preventive services and providing some compensation for skilled interventions for chronic conditions. Financial rewards for the physician, however, are currently far greater when the patient shows up in the office or emergency room needing hospitalization. Although ongoing care management and primary care can avoid most of the critical episodes that lead to hospital stays, the system of Medicare reimbursement has not incorporated the management of chronic conditions into standard Medicare coverage.

Who Decides?

In the original Medicare legislation, Congress defined about fifty-five benefit categories, with certain exclusions and limits, but did not compose a complete list.[8] Instead, seeking to provide flexibility for health security as well as fiscal security against unlimited claims, Congress stipulated that covered items and services in general must be "reasonable and necessary."

The purpose of coverage is defined as the "treatment and diagnosis of illness or injury." This language, which reflects the acute, episodic focus of medical care forty years ago, is at the root of the challenge of incorporating modern geriatric medicine into Medicare. Under existing guidelines, preventive and primary care is essentially excluded; legislation or formal rules are required to cover specific preventive services as exceptions.

Congress delegated administrative authority for implementation of Medicare coverage to the Health Care Financing Administration (HCFA, now CMS, the Centers for Medicare and Medicaid Services) within the Department of Health and Human Services. In turn, CMS contracts with insurance companies, called "intermediaries," for Part A and "carriers" for Part B. HCFA did not develop a formal process by which to specify medical necessity because the agency expected contractors and providers to fix most of the details and resolve disputes locally, as they did already for commercial health insurance. As a result, Medicare policy is largely dictated by local Medical Review Policies devised by regional claims processors, which produce a wide variation in standards across the country.[9] CMS rarely has a reason, or sufficient funding, to review these local policies to determine whether they are uniform, reasonable, and necessary.

Legal challenges of coverage decisions in the mid-1980s put pressure on the agency to develop guidelines for a uniform national policy for coverage, but most of these efforts have been derailed by for-profit stakeholders (led by the medical device industry) alarmed at the prospect of centralized coverage decisions that might reduce their markets.[10] Although various bodies advise CMS, like the current Medicare Coverage Advisory Committee (MCAC), established in 1999, rule making continues to be a confusing process of uncertain authority and energy. National coverage determinations are rarely supported by a formal process that courts will recognize. Immediate decisions by intermediaries define Medicare coverage based on rules that conform to practices in the private insurance industry.

Although Medicare has modernized incrementally, many coverage and payment decisions seem arbitrary. Why, for example, is prostate screening covered by Medicare, while other preventive services, such as heart-failure management, are not? Why are people with end-stage renal disease fully covered by Medicare, regardless of age, when those under age sixty-five lucky enough to receive a kidney transplant automatically lose coverage for follow-up care afterward? Why is a physician not paid for taking the time to talk to an eighty-five-year-old cancer patient, answer the family's questions, and determine whether a particularly painful or risky procedure is appropriate—yet is paid well for giving chemotherapy drugs, whether appropriate or not? Why are some experimental procedures covered and others not? Why can some people get an experimental procedure covered by going through an appeals process while others are unable to get the same procedure covered, either because they do not appeal or because their case is decided by a judge in a different region?

Decisions about Medicare coverage for technological innovations are also based on the "reasonable and necessary" standard, but there are no explicit criteria for defining what this means. For example, in 2003 CMS decided to provide coverage for three invasive, high-cost procedures—lung-volume reduction surgery, implantable cardioverter defibrillators, and left-ventricular assist devices—at a projected total cost of between $1.3 and $11.4 billion. A different process was used to reach a final decision for each of these procedures; but in all three cases the decision was based on an exhaustive analysis of available scientific data, with the Coverage and Analysis Group of CMS evaluating the reported benefits and health outcomes. However, the evaluation process is not based on explicit criteria such as the use of a minimum cost-effectiveness ratio, which would require CMS to consider both the potential benefits and costs of a new technology or procedure. Congressional action is necessary if the criterion of "reasonable and necessary" is to be refined to include considerations of cost and appropriateness.

This system operates fine as long as one remains healthy. Among those with severe illness or disability, dissatisfaction is widespread.[11] A patient may face unexpected payment obstacles in the course of medical care, which providers will attempt to resolve with varying degrees of effort and consideration. These efforts may be frustrated by the decisions of intermediaries that determine the limits of coverage according to their own definitions of medical necessity.

Physicians may face requirements of preapproval for treatment, denial of payment, and coverage gaps that impede the continuity of care. Professional autonomy is eroded as procedures get bundled into groups for reimbursement reasons, then restricted to eliminate "excess" profit. CMS has acted nationwide to reduce payments to doctors and hospitals as a way to curtail growing costs when there is no political will to increase taxes to cover Medicare. The pharmaceutical industry has proved to be a more powerful political force than doctors, requiring, for example, that the new prescription drug law prohibit Medicare from negotiating lower prices for beneficiaries or using cost-effectiveness research to support coverage decisions.

The policy vacuum at the center is a critical issue in Medicare coverage. Indecision over the definition of medical necessity (or "demonstrated medical effectiveness" or "medical benefit and added value") prevails because agency interests do not want to open nor commercial interests close new territories of costly medical services. Every single Medicare decision is a political one, played out in the tension between providers and corporate financial interests and the government's commitment to cutting expenditures and reducing taxes. In this environment, a needed comprehensive restructuring of Medicare seems impossible.

OUT-OF-POCKET EXPENSES

Many decisions about medical necessity are still based on the patient's pocketbook. As in the early 1960s, the elderly and their families bear a heavy burden of medical costs. The gaps in Medicare coverage limit its ability to protect older adults and their families from impoverishment due to medical expenses, especially as more care is required for chronic disorders needing out-of-hospital treatment and coordination of services in community settings.

Out-of-pocket health-care spending for seniors is now already higher than it was in the years before Medicare. The premiums, deductibles, and copayments associated with Medicare and Medicare supplemental insurance consume a significant portion of seniors' income. In 1965 (before Medicare), older adults spent 19 percent of their personal income on health care.[12] In 1968, the percentage dropped to 11 percent. In 2002, the typical senior on Medicare spent 22 percent of income on health care, an average of $3,757 per year.[13] For those in poor health, 10 percent of Medicare beneficiaries pay an average of $9,174 or more out of pocket. More than $9,000 per year obviously has greater impact on lower-income households.

Out-of-pocket health-care costs are growing substantially for all Americans. Medicine that can do more costs more. All insurers are passing on more costs to the patient. Although Medicare has significantly lightened the burden of some health-care costs, such as inpatient hospital care, older citizens still pay high costs in many other areas of health care, including prescription drugs and hospital copayments. The Medicare reform ideas of many Republican leaders include increasing copayments by patients in the belief that doing so will reduce government costs and make patients more discerning consumers.

Although Medicare and Social Security have significantly reduced poverty rates among the elderly, median incomes remain low. Median family income for Medicare beneficiaries in 1999 was $24,817, with 40 percent living on incomes below 200 percent of the federal poverty level.[14] Rates of poverty or near poverty increase with age, especially for women and minorities. Health-care costs that older adults are unable to pay are frequently passed on to younger generations, either directly, as adult children help their parents financially, or indirectly, as savings are depleted that otherwise might have supported education and other opportunities for children and grandchildren.

SUPPLEMENTAL INSURANCE

Inadequate Medicare coverage encourages a market for supplemental health insurance. In 1999 this gap was filled by employer-sponsored coverage for 33 percent of beneficiaries, by private policies (called Medigap) for 27 percent, and by Medicaid for 11 percent.[15] Retirement health insurance is offered almost exclusively by large firms with two hundred or more employees. Of these, only about one-fourth offer such a benefit, and these tend to be the largest firms, with five thousand or more employees.[16] Employer plans, which typically pay over half the cost of the monthly premium, offer the best deal for seniors, but the number and extent of employer-sponsored plans declined through the 1990s; and a current survey shows a continuing increase in premiums, cost sharing, and benefit caps.[17]

Premiums for all private health insurance policies have been increasing at double-digit rates. Medigap insurance, however, poses a special financial burden. Although neither Medigap nor managed care fully protects patients from high out-of-pocket costs,[18] the choice between managed-care plans or the ten standard options for Medigap insurance can make a considerable financial difference, depending on age and health.[19] Unfortunately, there is no easy way to determine the right choice. By choosing to rely on traditional Medicare and paying a minimum premium for Part B, the elderly risk exposure to significant coverage gaps; by choosing a Medigap policy, they risk spending $400 to $20,000 per year for coverage that may not be needed. For a person on a low, fixed income with uncertain health, this can be a treacherous decision.

FLEXIBLE FINANCING

To ensure Medicare's future effectiveness requires a flexible system capable of changing coverage and payment rules as technology and medicine advance, while also ensuring fairness. Expanding the notion of medical necessity beyond acute episodes to incorporate chronic conditions and long-term attention to functional capacity and health maintenance requires allowing direct decision making by physicians rather than reliance on arbitrary rules. Resolving the competing ideals of flexibility and standardization is a challenge not often voiced in the political debates over Medicare, which typically concentrate on cost control.

What are the alternatives to congressional micromanagement and irrational Medicare rules? How can we standardize decisions while maintaining flexibility? Reforming the present system will require overcoming ideological agendas and looking for models that support modern geriatric medicine. Managed care is part of the answer. Done right, managed care can expand coverage and provide the flexibility to coordinate care for complex chronic illness.

Making Managed Care Work

Medicare began experimenting with managed-care contracting in 1982 but only formalized the process as a standard option in 1997, with Medicare+Choice. Contractors who participate are required to provide all benefits covered by traditional Medicare; in fact, the expectation was that they offer more benefits with lower cost to the patient (cost-sharing) and sometimes zero premiums to increase enrollment. CMS pays the contractors an average premium that combines expected costs for Parts A and B of Medicare. BBA 1997 expanded the range of potential contracts to include not only insurers but also hospitals and other provider organizations willing to accept the risk of prepayment in exchange for providing guaranteed medical benefits. This program held out the promise of good managed care with the flexibility of prepaid systems. Some were successful; many were not.

One of the first problems to emerge in the system was huge losses by provider organizations that miscalculated the risks involved. This problem was not restricted to Medicare but reverberated through the whole managed-care marketplace in the late 1990s with a rash of failures.[20] Eliminating the insurer as an intermediary by contracting directly with doctors and hospitals no longer looks like a viable strategy.

The original enthusiasm for capitation—the idea of prepayment for health care—has diminished significantly but not completely vanished. Integrated systems of finance and delivery, like Kaiser Permanente, which operates on a large scale and has experience in managing the health of elderly patients, continue to do well under capitation and are able to provide coordinated, flexible care consistent with the principles of geriatric medicine. Despite a backlash against provider risk contracting, in places where it works, it gives providers greater autonomy over decisions in patient care, since they are bearing the financial risk themselves.[21]

Alarmed by numerous tales of denial of care, restricted networks, and unreliable benefits, the public has become increasingly skeptical of managed care; but this does not need to be the case. Under the right circumstances and with the right expertise and motives, managed care can accomplish the goals of coordinated and multidisciplinary care that are at the heart of good geriatric medicine. Direct contracting with provider-sponsored organizations looks like the most successful way to manage care, but the smaller population base that most group practices have for accepting financial risk is precarious. Once again, we see that a broad base to spread the insurance risk is essential. Contracting with an insurer to manage risk adds the problem of third-party decision making over medical necessity and limits of coverage, which can be frustrating for both physician and patient.

Of course, it is not always bad to limit expensive services. Overtreatment can be as dangerous as undertreatment, given the risks of side effects from some diagnostic tests as well as actual medical interventions. Some researchers have shown that traditional Medicare, which does not set limits on physician visits, tests, or treatments, creates an incentive for overtreatment.[22] Without proper care management, patients may submit themselves to unnecessarily expensive, uncomfortable, and potentially risky diagnostic procedures and treatments.

Capitation can work well or badly depending on the motives, expertise, and resources of those providing care. This is why it is so important to create and use reliable measures of quality that consumers can understand. Although some Medicare HMOs provide good care and elicit high consumer satisfaction ratings, consumer satisfaction is not the only or even the best measure of quality. There is evidence that people in Medicare HMOs do not receive as many expensive services as those in traditional Medicare,[23] but it is hard to know if this situation results in better or worse outcomes, since overuse of services is as big a quality problem as underuse. Other areas of care also show differences. A singular study in 2002, comparing primary care in HMOs with that in traditional Medicare, found that nine of eleven indicators favored traditional Medicare.[24] Lower out-of-pocket costs were considered an advantage to HMOs for many patients. No difference appeared in measures of preventive counseling.

For convalescence or care at the end of life, basic services such as home care are not often covered by traditional Medicare and are harder to obtain. Capitated programs are not restricted by these Medicare rules and may offer more of these "high-touch" services while restricting unnecessary "high-tech" services. In all, the real question to ask in determining good care should be not "What does Medicare cover?" but "What does the patient really need?"

POSITIVE FEATURES OF CAPITATION

Theoretically, prospective payment produces an incentive to concentrate on preventive care. In the 1960s and 1970s, research about the importance of preventive medical interventions and lifestyle changes began to draw attention, and primary care and preventive medicine became standard practice. As a result, commercial insurance began to cover primary care for the first time. Perhaps the most dramatic application of the primary-care concept was applied to patient care in large, multispecialty, not-for-profit HMOs, including the Kaiser Permanente system, Group Health, Harvard Community Health Plans, and Health Partners and other plans in Minnesota. These group and staff-model HMOs (where doctors are paid by salary, not fee-for-service) have been real innovators, though they were not widely understood or accepted in the medical world when they began.

With a capitated system, the health plan has an incentive to keep enrollees healthy in order to reduce their need for costly treatment. For the younger, working population, this means investments in such measures as primary care, screening tests, prenatal and well-child care, and patient education. For an aging population, it also involves active, collaborative management of chronic conditions.

When done well, managed care offers a personalized and comprehensive approach to care, potentially giving enrollees access to interdisciplinary teams, primary care, home care, and continuity of care, all with an emphasis on prevention. By transferring the risk of health-care costs to the providers of care, capitation in Medicare contracting could encourage a flexible, efficient use of resources at the point of service without uniform mandates and volumes of national regulations. Unfortunately, managed care has failed to work reliably in practice.

NEGATIVE FEATURES OF CAPITATION

Capitation may encourage innovative measures to manage care, but a simpler means of increasing profits in the private marketplace is simply to avoid enrolling high-risk individuals who are likely to need more expensive health care. Risk selection is a threat to the effectiveness of Medicare managed-care contracts. Numerous studies confirm that M+C insurers attracted healthier Medicare beneficiaries who didn't need expensive specialized care,[25] but many of these beneficiaries left managed care if the company had very restrictive limits on specialists and returned to traditional Medicare when expensive treatments became necessary.[26] The M+C program therefore did not save money for Medicare.[27] Fragmenting the Medicare risk pool into diverse private plans increases the insurance risk, so that large profits are necessary to encourage plans to participate at all. As a result, CMS finds itself in the dilemma of trying to cut costs yet also encourage widespread participation. The new Medicare Advantage program that replaces M+C tries to address this by risk adjustment—paying more for sicker patients—but the marketplace pressures to limit expenses remain, especially for investor-owned companies.

According to interviews conducted for a Commonwealth Fund field report, corporate managed care is under tremendous pressure from Wall

Street to perform, and Medicare contracts received a low recommendation from investment analysts.[28] After 1999, hundreds of M+C plans withdrew from the program or dropped coverage for certain areas, leaving millions of beneficiaries without coverage other than traditional Medicare.[29] M+C plans also reduced benefits, increased cost sharing, changed their networks of providers, and added complex restrictions on access to care, thereby creating an environment of uncertainty and dissatisfaction for beneficiaries.[30] One study found that Medicare HMOs routinely changed coverage rules and denied care they are required by law to provide, including emergency and urgent care.[31] Congressional action in 2000 to increase payments to M+C contractors did little to improve the situation.[32]

Only about 12 percent of Medicare beneficiaries were enrolled in M+C plans in 2004, and the predictions for the new Medicare Advantage program are uncertain. Participation is concentrated in a few states, mostly in the West, where contractors have more experience with managed care and where over 40 percent of beneficiaries may be enrolled; other states have few or no options for managed care. Like managed care in general, M+C and Medicare Advantage are almost nonexistent in rural areas. Increasing payments to contractors is not likely to resolve the severe regional disparities.[33]

ORGANIZING FOR SUCCESS

One possible reason for the failure of so many managed Medicare plans is their lack of understanding of good geriatric care. Coordinated, interdisciplinary care management requires substantial infrastructure and experience. Good information systems are required to provide consistent information to multiple specialists, thus reducing redundant tests and the risks of missing important diagnoses, allergies, or other clinical facts. Proactive communication with patients and families is also required to educate patients about managing chronic conditions such as diabetes and heart failure and to head off exacerbations of illness and avoid hospitalization. When hospitalization does occur, a well-functioning geriatric team is necessary to reduce the chances of complications and ease the transition home or to rehabilitation.

These practical steps, which can be called "prospective" or "anticipatory care," require geriatric medicine experts. Many managed Medicare plans do not use geriatric models or geriatricians, in part because their strategy is to focus on the younger elderly (sixty-five- to seventy-five-year-olds) who are less likely to have complex health-care needs. Even among this population, some will develop conditions requiring geriatric management; but the people who benefit most from good managed care are those over seventy-five. The lack of care management raises concerns about the wisdom of more loosely structured organizations such as "health plans" linked only by an insurance company taking on managed-care Medicare contracts. With no infrastructure for care coordination or information exchange, it is difficult to sustain an effective quality of care, and costs can quickly outpace contracted Medicare payments.

How Can Managed Medicare Succeed?

Efforts to solve the many problems in the marketplace for Medicare managed care should always be compared to traditional Medicare and other choices that might be made to reduce costs and administrative burdens and achieve equivalent outcomes for beneficiaries. With a few exceptions, the instability of the managed Medicare program shows little success in improving coverage or flexibility or reducing costs. Insurers' attempts to remedy the situation involve a number of extremely complex approaches that may be neither reasonable or necessary.

RISK SELECTION

Medicare managed-care contractors have refined the practice of risk selection—the process of seeking out the healthiest patients, who will not need much care, while discouraging enrollment by those who are likely to need expensive care. (Ironically, it is the patients with the most complex problems who are likely to benefit most from the flexibility of good managed care.) M+C contractors did attract a healthier subset of the Medicare population, but the result is apparently not due to marketing alone. Individuals with more complex health-care needs seem to prefer the more secure, though spotty, coverage of traditional Medicare rather than risk the uncertainties of the private market.[34]

One alternative to excluding high-risk patients from coverage is to charge a higher premium for their care. The idea of risk-adjusted premiums has existed for decades. In theory, compensation from higher premiums encourages commercial insurers to accept higher-risk clients and manage their care appropriately. The idea is really no different from the practice of experience rating in the normal commercial insurance market.

A risk-adjusted premium for Medicare is another form of experience rating, whereby a commercial insurer essentially charges the government a higher premium for accepting a higher risk. The higher payments are intended to attract health plans to enroll Medicare Advantage (managed care) patients.

The risk-adjustment system currently being implemented, called the Principal Inpatient Diagnostic Cost Group (PIP-DCG), attempts to correct some of the inadequacies of the previous adjustment system. However, to develop a precise method of risk adjustment, accounting for each patient's risk factors, would require a monumental effort and calculations of Byzantine complexity. A clear understanding of the goal suggests the result would be nothing more than the prediction of a fair price for sustained costs. "Like so much else about the U.S. health system," one analyst concludes, "it seems an astonishingly complex way to achieve some straightforward policy goals."[35] Many experts believe that risk selection will continue to lead to healthier beneficiaries enrolling in Medicare Advantage private plans and less healthy beneficiaries being funneled into traditional Medicare.[36] These patients may well pay more out of pocket because private plans are allowed to impose such charges. Medicare could be better served and strengthened by resisting the market pressures to fragment the sick from the currently healthy and maintain a common payment mechanism in prepaid care, while keeping risk adjustment for traditional Medicare.

CONSUMER INFORMATION

A second major area of concern in managed-care marketing is the inability of consumers to evaluate alternative plans and select one that matches their anticipated needs. A similar problem in the market for Medigap insurance was addressed in 1990 by legislation that required private policies to conform to a set of ten standard benefit packages. The standardization did not completely resolve problems of selection or fulfill the need for consumer information, but it did improve price competition because it made it easier for buyers to compare different companies' policies.[37] The issue is more complicated for Medicare private plans because in many markets there may be only one plan offered, and the choice is between an HMO on the one hand and traditional Medicare, supplemented by a private Medigap policy, on the other.

Health-care consumers should be well informed and involved in their care decisions, but expecting them to be so well informed that they apply market pressure for efficiency and innovation, as would occur in the ideal market, is asking far too much. The many problems with the current model of consumer-driven health care raise grave doubts that markets of this sort can give us the health system we want.

LOSS OF COVERAGE

Patient protection has become a major concern in recent years, following abuses and complaints in the managed-care marketplace. Most regulation occurs at the state level. For Medicare, the primary concern is to provide adequate access and coordinated services for those with chronic conditions. CMS can operate most effectively by standardizing diverse state laws for credentials, access to specific services, requirements for an adequate network of providers, quality benchmarks, and, perhaps most important from a national perspective, uniform data reporting on quality measures.[38]

People on Medicare who lose HMO coverage are in a precarious position when they are forced to return to traditional Medicare. In most states, people are guaranteed the ability to buy Medigap policies only during very limited periods of time, such as within three months after being involuntarily terminated from an HMO.[39] If an individual is dropped from an HMO and does not buy a Medigap policy in that time, the chance to buy an affordable, preferred policy may be lost. This is especially likely when the person has a preexisting health condition like heart disease or diabetes. AARP sells Medigap policies to people with preexisting conditions, but these may still be prohibitively expensive.

INTERFACE WITH LONG-TERM CARE

Coverage for care in a skilled-nursing facility (SNF) or at home has always been constrained by definitions aiming to delimit episodes with a clear beginning and end and stipulating numerous exclusions, in a manner that follows closely the practice of private insurance. Unfortunately, this attitude neglects the real needs of elderly and disabled individuals. The private market for insurance has never been very willing to apply itself to the losing proposition of long-term care. Although this failure suggests that a solution should be achieved through social insurance, with a system like Medicare, the topic of long-term care is hardly ever raised in serious policy discussions because the potential cost makes the issue unpopular and apparently intractable.

This does not need to be the case. In many other countries where life expectancy is greater than in the United States, access to long-term care services is universal. Germany enacted a universal system for long-term care insurance in 1994, to replace its means-tested program, which was similar to Medicaid. Experience there has shown that a modest 1.7 percent payroll tax has managed to support a sustainable system that also supports informal caregivers.[40] While costs may be greater in the United States, success in countries as diverse as Sweden and Japan demonstrates that an affordable solution is possible, given the political will to achieve it.

The supposed overuse of SNF and home care, reflected in escalating costs, caused Congress in BBA 1997 to apply prospective-payment systems to these areas of care. The results were a severe reduction in reimbursement levels and the closure of many facilities and home-care businesses. Concerns over rising expenditures are justified, but coordination of care across Medicare and Medicaid paid domains would reduce costs while maintaining a higher standard of care. The types of burdens faced now by Medicare beneficiaries are suggested in the following story, which reflects only one of the many denials of care resulting from strict definitions of medical necessity.

Mr. Steven Noble is a sixty-five-year-old independent-minded farmer in the Midwest. Fifteen years ago, he was paralyzed in a tractor accident and is now unable to move his legs or arms. Fortunately, he has a loving wife and a big, supportive family nearby. Because of the severity of his disability, Mr. Noble is eligible for home-health care covered by Medicare. A home-health nurse comes several days a week to bathe him and turn him over so that he will not develop dangerous bed sores. One day, the nurse tells his wife she can no longer come to their home to provide services, as Mr. Noble is no longer eligible under Medicare. Mrs. Noble is dismayed. Her husband's condition has not changed, and she is not in great health herself. She certainly cannot give her husband all the care he needs by herself.

The home-health nurse points to the specially designed van for people with disabilities that sits in the family's driveway. "Does Mr. Noble ever go into that van?" she asks.

"Once a week, the family puts him into a cart and brings him to Wal-Mart or the park," Mrs. Noble answers, expecting the nurse to congratulate her for keeping her husband involved in his family's life.

"Well, then, he is not homebound. If he can leave the house, Medicare will not pay for his home health care," the nurse says.[41] Mr. Noble lost his home care coverage.

Because of examples like this, in February 2001 the definition of *home-bound* was expanded to include trips to receive health-care treatment and other trips that are "infrequent or of a relatively short duration," including "any absence for the purpose of attending a religious service."[42]

ALL-INCLUSIVE CARE

Long-term care is clearly an integral part of modern geriatric medicine and cannot be separated from good medical care. Because the principles of care coordination and multidisciplinary teams are vital when treating frail elders, good geriatric medicine acknowledges no dividing line between acute and chronic or long-term care. What is vital to high-quality, patient-centered care is continuity. Traditional Medicare's disjointed payment system fails to support this kind of appropriate care. The results of PACE (Program of All-Inclusive Care for the Elderly) demonstrate that capitated payments can allow the flexibility necessary for coordination of care. PACE offers a good model for financing flexible, coordinated care management that covers both acute and chronic conditions.

In PACE, patients and their physicians are not limited by exclusions in Medicare coverage. The capitation fee, combining Medicare and Medicaid reimbursement, eliminates cost shifting. It reduces overall costs and leads to significantly better outcomes, including fewer nurse visits, hospital admissions, and hospital and nursing-home days as well as improvement in functional status, quality of life, satisfaction with care, and socialization.[43] Chapter 4 discusses PACE in more detail.

Because Medicaid covers two-thirds of all nursing-home residents and pays for nearly half of all nursing-home expenditures,[44] providers have a substantial incentive to collaborate with Medicare in caring for the frail elderly in a way that keeps these patients out of nursing homes, improves their health, personalizes care, and reduces costs. Although it does not pay for long-term care, Medicare does pay for medical care for many recipients of long-term care. Nearly one-third of all Medicare spending goes to the 13 percent of beneficiaries with significant long-term care needs, and beneficiaries who need long-term care cost on average more than three times as much as those who do not.[45]

Since Medicare and Medicaid together cover so many older people, a federal social-insurance plan that combines acute and long-term care would make a lot of sense. PACE is small compared to the needs of elders across the nation, but the model of care it represents may gradually lead to broader acceptance of the idea of combining the Medicare and

Medicaid components of coverage for the frail elderly to avoid cost-shifting and encourage care management and continuity.

MEDICARE AND MEDICAID

Six and a half million people, or about 16 percent of each program's enrollment, are covered jointly by Medicare and Medicaid. These patients are known as "dual eligibles." For the majority of older citizens requiring long-term care, Medicare and Medicaid work together clumsily, fragmenting options for care and complicating the system for providers, patients, and families.

Dual eligibles tend to require expensive medical services, especially long-term care, and use a disproportionate share of each program's funds. In 1997, they accounted for about 28 percent of Medicare spending and 35 percent of Medicaid spending nationwide. Two and a half million of these dual eligibles may obtain full coverage for both Medicare and Medicaid benefits.[46] Many others are not eligible for full Medicaid benefits but receive financial assistance in meeting Medicare's cost-sharing requirements. For moderately low-income seniors, Medicaid supplements Medicare benefits by paying the Part B premium, along with some deductibles and copayments. For those with lower incomes, Medicaid may also pay for services Medicare does not cover, like long-term care in the home or nursing home.

Medicare and Medicaid are both government-run health-insurance programs, but they are dissimilar in many ways. The two programs come out of different worldviews. Medicare is based on a social-contract model and enrolls all older citizens and people with disabilities, regardless of income. Medicaid is a means-tested welfare program that enrolls only low-income adults and children. The two programs also differ in the following ways:

> *Coverage rules.* Unlike Medicare, Medicaid is a comprehensive health-insurance program that pays for prescription drugs, long-term care, and other services Medicare does not cover, including eyeglasses, hearing aids, and dental care.

> *Financing and administration.* Different levels of government finance and administer the two programs. Each state has flexibility in implementing its Medicaid benefits package and eligibility criteria. State criteria are widely variable and may change from year to year. Medicare criteria for medical necessity may also vary according to the policies

of regional intermediaries and carriers. Consolidation is no simple matter.

Reimbursement rates for providers. Medicaid tends to reimburse providers at lower rates than Medicare. As a result, most physicians are willing to treat Medicare patients, but far fewer treat Medicaid patients.

Because of the different structures of these two large programs, it is difficult to coordinate their administration. Often, it is unclear which program will pay for which services and at what rate. Recently, some federal and state policy makers have become interested in studying exactly how Medicare and Medicaid work together in different states, hoping to identify ways to save money and improve the coordination of care.[47] Certainly, overcoming fragmentation in care for this vulnerable population promises benefits for a number of stakeholders, including beneficiaries, providers, administrators, and taxpayers.

CHAPTER 7

Why Sixty-five?

The Case for Lowering the Age of Medicare Eligibility

Today, most sixty-five-year-olds are healthy, active, and productive. Nevertheless, sixty-five is the accepted age for retirement in the United States and the age at which eligibility for Social Security benefits and Medicare coverage begins. Does this policy make sense? What would be the effect of changing the age of eligibility for Social Security and Medicare? What is the rationale for the chronological link between Social Security and Medicare?

People with chronic conditions can age successfully if they get the medical care they need in time to avoid serious complications. Presently, many people neglect their health needs in their early sixties in order to postpone treatment until age sixty-five, when they become eligible for Medicare.[1] Assuring health-care access to this group might reduce overall costs and improve the health for those at higher risk.

Sixty-five is an arbitrary retirement age chosen originally in 1889 by Germany's chancellor Bismarck, who established old-age pensions for industrial and agrarian workers, artisans, and servants.[2] Of course, in 1889 only a small percentage of the population survived to age sixty-five, but in many countries it remains the age at which people traditionally retire and become eligible for benefit programs for the elderly.

This tradition is now subject to reexamination. Congress recently chose to postpone eligibility for Social Security to age sixty-seven over the next twenty years. From the perspective of modern geriatric medicine, it makes sense to consider lowering the age for Medicare eligibility while raising the age for Social Security.

People aged fifty-five through sixty-four have a higher risk than younger people for developing chronic conditions and cancer.[3] For this intermediate age group, comprehensive health insurance could ensure access to medical care and help prevent major complications and premature death. Because they are more likely than younger workers to experience employment gaps necessitated by caregiving responsibilities or their own health problems, people in this intermediate age group may lose their employee health insurance just when they need it most.

Many people who retire early do so because of a decline in their overall health. A recent study found self-reported health status is the single most important predictor of work status for those in their fifties. More than half of the men and one-third of the women who stop working before reaching the Social Security early-retirement age of sixty-two report that health limits their capacity to work.[4] At present these people are not eligible for Medicare unless they can establish a qualifying disability, and they find it hard to buy individual health insurance because of their pre-existing conditions.

The availability of guaranteed health insurance through Medicare would be unlikely to promote widespread early retirement. One analysis suggests that only an additional 1.1 percent of the cohort aged fifty-five to sixty-four would choose early retirement because of the offer of health insurance.[5] Yet for those in poor health and who are already disposed to retire or reduce their work commitments, health insurance could make a significant difference in health and income security.

Arguing to lower the age for Medicare eligibility and raise the age for Social Security runs against the traditional thinking about these two programs and is bound to meet resistance, but the proposal is worth thinking about. The potential for improving the quality of life for those aged fifty-five to sixty-four is significant. Early care management would also help to reduce complications and costs for this group as they age. Keeping the "young-old" healthy and working can be good for individuals, good for the sustainability of the nation's old-age health and pension systems, and good for the overall prosperity of our society and economy.

Special Needs of Older Midlife Adults

Adults aged fifty-five to sixty-four, like younger people, depend primarily on employment-based health coverage. They are more likely to be uninsured if they have low income or a disability, belong to a minority group, or are single.[6] Although young adults have the highest rate of uninsurance,[7] older adults are more likely to be separated from the workforce through disabilities (11 percent) or retirement (24 percent). They are also more likely to rate their health as fair or poor. Those with poorer health are more likely to be uninsured.

The uninsured are more likely to report problems accessing health care, more likely to delay seeking care, and more likely to experience avoidable hospitalizations for such conditions as diabetes, hypertension, and bleeding ulcers.[8] Insured adults are more likely to keep up to date with preventive exams such as routine physical exams, Pap smears, mammograms, and prostate exams.[9] Lack of health insurance later in life is more likely to have serious consequences.

Chronic Conditions and Modern Medicine

In general, the incidence of disease and the associated mortality increase steadily through middle age and the young-old years and then increase more steeply as people enter their mid-seventies and early eighties. According to the 1997 National Health Interview Survey of adults aged 55 to 64, 28 percent had a disability that limited their daily activities, compared with 19 percent of those aged 45 to 54 and 10 percent of those aged 18 to 44.[10] Similarly, rates of chronic conditions such as arthritis and hypertension are noticeably higher at age 45 and higher still at age 55.

Disorders that become more common in late middle age and benefit from early detection and management include hypertension, diabetes, breast cancer, osteoporosis, and coronary heart disease. These are discussed in more detail below. Early detection of such conditions can improve care management and prevent disability, leading to more years of quality life.

HYPERTENSION

When individuals with borderline hypertension (defined as above 130 over 85) are included, about half of all people over sixty-five have hypertension.[11] The rate for adults aged fifty to fifty-nine is about 40 percent.[12]

Reducing blood pressure significantly decreases the risk of serious conditions, including cardiovascular death, congestive heart failure, kidney failure, and stroke. Hypertension is usually best treated with a combination of lifestyle changes and medication. Medications are effective, but side effects are highly variable. Close follow-up with a physician is important.

CORONARY HEART DISEASE

Risk factors for coronary heart disease include age, male gender, heredity (including race), smoking, high blood pressure, high cholesterol, physical inactivity, obesity, diabetes, and kidney failure. Although four out of five people who die of coronary heart disease are sixty-five or older,[13] steps could be taken to prevent or minimize disease earlier in the life span.

Coronary heart disease presents one of the clearest economic arguments for lowering Medicare's eligibility age. If controllable risk factors are not managed earlier in life, people are likely to develop coronary heart disease after they become eligible for Medicare, requiring the expensive, invasive procedures of balloon angioplasty, implanting stents, or coronary artery bypass surgery. Medicare pays for these procedures. Many heart patients will also require medications for the rest of their lives. Significant savings could be achieved with anticipatory management of the conditions that put individuals at risk for coronary artery disease, thus reducing hospitalizations and avoiding expensive surgery.

DIABETES

Type 2 diabetes is increasing in prevalence. Across all age groups, prevalence increased 33 percent nationally between 1990 and 1998. Among those aged fifty to fifty-nine it increased 31 percent. Almost 10 percent of people in their fifties reported in 1998 that they had been diagnosed with diabetes.[14]

Diabetes treatment aims to normalize blood glucose levels, thereby reducing the risk of cardiovascular disease, stroke, kidney failure, blindness, and circulatory problems that can necessitate limb amputation.[15] There is a lot at stake in identifying diabetes early and treating it aggressively. The best results are achieved with an interdisciplinary team working intensively with the patient and family. Intensive support can help individuals to change their diet and increase activity. Such lifestyle changes can reduce and sometimes even eliminate the need for medication. Most diabetics, however, need treatment such as insulin several times a day with frequent blood tests at home. The individual with diabetes needs to be well educated about the disease and must participate in self-care and monitoring. Good management of diabetes can make the difference between active, productive aging and severe disability.

Adequate health insurance is a key element in managing diabetes. Uninsured diabetics are more likely than those with insurance to be hospitalized for treatment of complications,[16] which can require expensive medical care and shorten life. Managed-care organizations are now commonly using disease-management programs (diet and medication reminders, weight-loss support groups, early screenings for complications) to give special attention to diabetics, finding that investing time and energy early on saves money later.

BREAST CANCER

The risk of breast cancer increases with age. A woman's chance of being diagnosed with breast cancer is one out of 252 at age forty, one out of 68 at age fifty, one out of 35 at age sixty, and one out of 27 at age seventy.[17] Because early detection is critical in the treatment of breast cancer, all women require regular screening. A combination of regular mammography, breast exams by a physician, and breast self-examination is known to improve the chances of early detection.[18]

A recent Centers for Disease Control (CDC) report found that although the rate of overall screening among women, as recommended by the American Cancer Society, rose from 31 percent to 47 percent between 1990 and 1995, the use of appropriate breast-cancer screening remains low among several subgroups, including women with low income, less education, and no health insurance.[19] The 1997 National Health Interview Survey found that breast-cancer screening rates vary by insurance status: among women over age forty, 73 percent of insured women had had a mammogram within the last two years, compared to only 50 percent of uninsured women. According to another survey, the uninsured are more likely to die from breast cancer, even after controlling for other health problems. The uninsured are less likely to be screened and therefore are more likely to develop breast cancer that is diagnosed too late for effective treatment.[20]

OSTEOPOROSIS

Hip fractures result in approximately three hundred thousand hospital admissions each year in the United States and an estimated $9 billion in direct medical costs. Most of these fractures result from osteoporosis among women who experience accelerated bone loss after menopause. Measurement of bone mineral density (BMD) is the best tool available to assess postmenopausal osteoporotic fracture risk. In a CDC study, 93 percent of estrogen-deficient women with osteoporosis, as defined by BMD, were unaware of their condition.[21]

Awareness makes a difference, since osteoporosis can be treated with medication and improved nutrition. For the majority of women at risk for osteoporosis, maximum bone loss occurs in the years just after menopause, usually between ages fifty and sixty. These women are not eligible for Medicare at the time when screening and prevention could provide the greatest benefit.

RETIREMENT, CAREGIVING, AND WORK

The proposal to reduce Medicare eligibility to age fifty-five shows merit on its own account but would work best, with fewer costs and greater benefit to society, if considered in combination with raising the eligibility age for Social Security. As more individuals successfully manage chronic diseases, they will remain healthy enough to work and pay income taxes well into their seventies. Instead of receiving Social Security benefits, these citizens would continue to contribute to the Social Security fund by paying FICA taxes.

Are workers willing to retire later? When asked if they want to retire at age sixty-five, the answer of most Americans seems to be "Yes and no." Survey respondents repeatedly say they want to retire "young" from their primary career and stop working long hours, but they also say they would like to keep working in some capacity. In the Health and Retirement Study, over three-fourths of respondents reported they would prefer to reduce hours gradually rather than retire abruptly.[22] Yet the most common pattern of retirement from full-time work is complete retirement.

Why does this discrepancy exist between how and when people want to retire and what they actually do? The inflexibility of most jobs in the traditional labor market is largely responsible. For many people in their sixties, the demands of their own health and family caregiving are hard to coordinate with a full-time job.

An individual who takes time off from work to care for a spouse, parent, or other family member often jeopardizes his or her job. Increasingly, people fifty-five to sixty-five years old have living parents in their eighties or nineties who require family support. The Family and Medical Leave Act (FMLA) allows some employees to take twelve weeks of unpaid, insured leave to care for a relative, but this law applies to too few people and allows an insufficient length of time off work. Most older people die after a long period of functional decline and require home care and support for substantially longer than three months. A flexible work schedule over a longer period of time would be better in these situations.

The importance of caregiving to families and our economy should not be underestimated. Two out of five people over age seventy, and almost half of those over age eighty, need help with one or more daily activities. Most live in the community, cared for by family members who are not paid for their caregiving services. Almost three-quarters of the people caring for these elders are family members: 42 percent are their children, and 25 percent are spouses. These unpaid services are estimated to be worth $196 billion each year, an expense that would be borne by Medicaid if family caregivers were not willing and available to help. Caregiving is an issue of utmost importance to the baby boomers and their families. By 2030, some twenty-one million older adults may need help dealing with activity limitations.[23]

Lowering Medicare's eligibility age would not reduce the need for family caregiving, but it would allow more family members to care for others without the fear of losing their health insurance when they need it most. Because of the emotional and physical stresses of caring for a sick relative, it is especially important for caregivers to protect their own health.

REVITALIZING OLD AGE

Many people retire before they are ready because their employers push them toward retirement, often with the aim of hiring younger workers at lower salaries. This financial motive reinforces a silent but prevalent ageism. The rising costs of pension and health benefits have been a major disincentive against hiring or retaining older workers.

Under current Medicare rules, companies with twenty or more employees must provide primary health insurance to Medicare-eligible employees if they also insure younger employees. Making Medicare the primary insurance for all Medicare-eligible citizens, regardless of employment status, could both simplify Medicare's overly complex body of rules and provide an incentive for companies to retain older workers. With this change, company benefit plans or private supplemental plans could be coordinated with Medicare benefits.

If workers aged fifty-five to sixty-four did not need employer-based health insurance, they would make ideal candidates for jobs that are not full-time or long-term but require workers with years of experience. A Productive Aging Survey of the Commonwealth Fund found that 46 percent of the fifty-five to sixty-four-year-old population was not working, though almost half of those were willing and able to work.[24] Most baby boomers say they want to continue working in some capacity after they retire. With the decline in availability of reliable pensions, more will need to keep working. One AARP survey found that more than 70 percent of baby boomers planned to keep working after age sixty-five, at least part-time. Some need to continue working out of financial necessity, but more often they simply want to work.[25]

Successful aging is the process of growing old while maintaining the physical, mental, and psychological capacities to live a full and engaged life. Older individuals who remain in the workforce stay mentally alert longer than those who do not work or engage themselves intellectually on a daily basis. Self-efficacy, mastery, and having control over one's life are strong determinants of successful aging. Older people who earn a salary are often more in control of their financial lives than those who must live on savings and Social Security alone. Engagement in paid work, unpaid work, and social activities can improve the physical, mental, and psychological well-being of older adults.[26] Staying active in society is far easier if a person is physically healthy. The proposal advanced here to lower the age of Medicare eligibility is one way to ensure better health for a longer period of successful aging.

With continuing advances in medicine and the accelerated aging of the population as the baby boomers advance toward retirement, it is especially important to keep older people working as long as possible. Controlling chronic conditions with anticipatory care management often involves prescription medication to help midlife and older adults manage their chronic conditions. Medicare's new outpatient prescription drug coverage has the potential to improve access to needed medications, but there are many concerns about its features and structure. This topic is likely to be the focus of intense debate in the public arena and among policy makers. Chapter 9 addresses this issue.

CHAPTER 8

Insurance

Concepts and Changes

Medicare struggles with the often conflicting demands to assure access to an expanding array of medical advances, deal with growing concerns about quality of care, and contain costs. The program attempts to meet these demands by deciding what kinds of benefits are covered and how (and how much) to pay for them. Finance involves both where the money comes from and how it is spent. Although I briefly outline the sources of Medicare revenue below, my attention is occupied mostly with principles of allocation: how Medicare decides coverage and fees for care and the effect of these choices on the care that is delivered. As a physician, a taxpaying citizen, and a potential beneficiary of Medicare, I consider the ultimate goal to be improving Medicare's capacity to offer high-quality, modern geriatric medicine. Arriving at ideas for finance reform that further this goal will require an understanding of where we are and how we got here.

Social Insurance

By 1965, advances in medical technology were becoming more effective at keeping older people alive with diseases that were previously fatal. Advances in the treatment of pneumonia and heart attack, for example, represented significant progress for patients in their seventies. New treatment options were adding new pressures, however, by increasing the cost of insurance to cover the risk of needing care. From a financial perspective, the time was ripe for Medicare as a way to manage the extraordinary expenses of providing health care to a clearly vulnerable population.

Medicare is commonly viewed as the driver of today's health-care market; it contributes a significant portion of nearly every hospital's operating budget and accounts for nearly one-third of the average physician's revenue.[1] In 2003, Medicare paid for about 20 percent of all physician and clinical services, about 30 percent of hospital costs and home health care, and 25 percent of all durable medical equipment.[2]

Not all of the growth in medical innovation over the last several decades can be attributed to Medicare and the financial security it offers to patients and providers, but Medicare did spawn a new era of interest in hospital systems and brought a new sense of enterprise to health care. Medicare data have formed the basis for much important medical research. Medical training programs in hospitals receive a significant portion of their funding through Medicare. In the nonprofit sector, Blue Cross and Blue Shield were boosted as designated intermediaries for claims processing. Commercial insurers responded with supplementary health insurance that was much more affordable for companies to purchase for retirees. Private Medigap policies proliferated.

Medicare alone has never provided adequate assurance against the risk of financial and health losses; supplementary coverage has always been required. The gap between what is funded and what a patient needs is due not to inefficient administration but to constraints in the scope of the original legislation.

Most funding for Part A (hospital) insurance comes from a 2.9 percent payroll tax, split equally between worker and employer. An additional 12.4 percent, also split equally between worker and employer, pays for Social Security. Together these taxes make up the FICA (Federal Insurance Contributions Act) withholding on paychecks. A wage cap on the Medicare tax was eliminated in 1994, though a cap is still in effect for Social Security. Removing the cap increased the tax base for Medicare by fully taxing the compensation of higher-income workers.

Part B (supplementary medical insurance) is voluntary but nearly universal, with 95 percent of eligible beneficiaries participating. Individual premiums—a standard $66.60 per month in 2004—cover one-fourth of the costs, with the remaining three-fourths funded from general federal revenues (mostly income taxes). Beginning in 2007, the Part B premium will be higher for individuals with incomes above $80,000 per year. Medicare managed-care plans sometimes contract to cover Part B services with a zero premium from beneficiaries, though most now charge a premium.

Part D is the new prescription drug benefit enacted in the Medicare Prescription Drug Improvement and Modernization Act of 2003. (Part C was the former Medicare+Choice managed care option, now subsumed under Part D as Medicare Advantage.) It will begin paying for outpatient prescription drugs in January 2006. Enrollment will be voluntary, with the 2006 premium estimated at about $35 per month. The new benefit will not be available through traditional Medicare; beneficiaries who remain in the traditional fee-for-service program can enroll separately in a private prescription drug plan. The alternative is enrollment in an integrated Medicare Advantage plan that includes all Medicare-covered benefits, including prescription drugs.

FINANCING THE FUTURE

Increases in funding are likely to be necessary to sustain current or improved Medicare benefits in the future. Congress increased the payroll tax for the Part A hospital trust fund from 1.6 percent in 1965 to 2.9 percent in 1986. Funding for Part B supplementary insurance is more flexible. The premium is continually raised by incremental amounts to cover a standard one-fourth of total costs. The remaining amount, no matter how it grows, is automatically appropriated from the general tax fund. In total, payroll taxes cover about half, and tax revenues plus premiums cover the rest.

For workers, a tax rate of 1.45 percent (with the other half paid by the employer) to cover a major portion of health-care expenses after age sixty-five seems like a good bargain, and, indeed, support for Medicare is high even among younger workers. Confidence could erode, however, as the payroll tax system transfers funds directly from the young to the old without accumulating reserves for future needs. The intergenerational aspect of Medicare financing should make younger people interested in the direction of Medicare policies and the intense debates taking place over how to structure the program for future stability.

The future of health care is likely to be influenced by the steady erosion of good coverage under employer-based benefit plans and the increasing costs in the commercial market for insurance. The proportion of workers in private businesses with employer-sponsored coverage declined from 71 percent in the late 1970s to about 64 percent in the mid-1990s and to 61 percent in 2002.[3] During a few years of prosperity the percentage of workers covered actually increased, and the decline now seems to have leveled out. But employers are more worried about double-digit increases in premiums for health insurance than about any other concern and are progressively shifting costs to employees.[4] A small proportion of employers are reducing eligibility or dropping coverage altogether. Employee contributions toward health insurance premiums are growing, with many more people enrolled in high-deductible, employer-based insurance plans. This current trend is worrisome for the health security of a large part of the population.

Traditional Medicare is a relatively straightforward system compared to the complex and constantly changing array of copayments, deductibles, exclusions, and administrative hassles encountered in private insurance and the lapses in coverage and changes required with every new job. Current efforts to privatize Medicare threaten to destroy the character of the program as a dependable source of support. Do we really want to encumber Medicare with the kinds of uncertainty people face in the private market for health insurance, especially if poor health leads to exorbitant costs or unavailable coverage?

A lifelong investment in Medicare hospital insurance, funded by a moderate payroll tax and a low premium for supplementary insurance subsidized from general tax revenues, assures access to health care in later life without imposing a devastating financial burden. Although out-of-pocket expenses for some beneficiaries are already too high, and adjustments need to be made to spread the costs more evenly, Medicare provides health insurance that most older people would be unable to afford—or even to find—if they had to rely on the private insurance market. This is a relief to their families as well. Dramatic increases in the costs of Medigap policies indicate the difficulty of obtaining health insurance later in life. By guaranteeing equal access, Medicare also protects those with chronic illnesses and other health problems, who are charged much higher premiums in the private insurance market. The fundamental concepts behind insurance really do matter, and they matter more as we grow older.

THE EMERGENCE OF HEALTH INSURANCE

Although social-insurance programs such as Medicare and Social Security are sometimes criticized as socialist, they are modeled on private insurance schemes developed in the first half of the twentieth century. Health insurance does not have a long history in the United States or anywhere else. The success of the nonprofit "Blues"—Blue Cross, covering hospital expenses, and Blue Shield, covering physician expenses—served as a model for Medicare Parts A and B. In the 1980s, the Blues combined and began earnest competition with other commercial health plans, offering comprehensive coverage and gradually merging with the for-profit industry. Meanwhile, traditional Medicare is still based on a model of coverage derived from the earliest days of health insurance.

Like the early Blues, Medicare operates by community rating, by which a standard premium is applied to everyone, regardless of health or preexisting conditions. As a mandatory single-payer plan without competition, Medicare avoids the common problem of adverse selection, whereby healthier individuals who feel they are paying too much to insure their personal risks opt out, leaving in the system only those people who need more services and incur higher costs. Community rating is not possible in a competitive environment that allows individual choice. The pressure of trying to operate community-rated insurance in a competitive environment is what forced the Blues to change tactics and begin offering experience-rated insurance tailored to individual needs. Experience rating works well for the healthy, who use few services and enjoy low rates, but disastrously for the unhealthy, who must pay high rates or remain uninsured.

One way for community rating to survive in a competitive market is by risk selection, whereby insurers seek to enroll only healthier individuals. Medicare avoids this problem, too. First, Medicare is conceived as a system of social insurance that must cover everyone equally. The mission is accomplished by establishing a large risk pool that spreads the high costs of a few over a broad population base, including many people who will need little or no care. The will to provide equal access to all, combined with an inclusive system that calls on everyone to participate, is what makes social insurance work. This is Medicare's greatest strength. Efforts to privatize care may undermine the foundation on which Medicare is built.

Health security through a system of universal insurance gives value to all beneficiaries by assuring coverage. Reducing uncertainty is valuable in itself, whether or not the coverage is used. This is why people willingly buy other forms of insurance. In health care, funds are funneled from the healthy to the unhealthy in a very narrow stream. Recent figures, commonly repeated in the same proportions, show 5 percent of the population using over 50 percent of health-care resources, and 50 percent using over 95 percent.[5] This leaves half the population using less than 5 percent of health-care resources. Similar figures apply to the older Medicare population, with a concentration of expenditures in the last year of life and especially during the last month.[6] How readily we accept this channeling of resources depends on how fully we accept the idea of a legitimate social contract, in which many individuals agree to share the risks and pay the costs for universal access to a vital good.

By 1950, private pension plans and Social Security, accident and health insurance (led by workers' compensation), and state-run unemployment insurance were all accepted forms of social insurance. A new idea of social cooperation, by contract, was becoming evident for the working population. Early union welfare plans, based on contribution systems, have been largely superseded by insurance with defined benefits. Rather than accumulate like a savings account, an insurance premium pays for security from risk among a defined group. Not everyone obtains material benefits from insurance, but everyone does enjoy an increased sense of security.

There is a tendency to think of insurance as a little like a savings account, however, and a stable membership over time helps guarantee regular contributions. Stability is one reason why Medicare is such a popular program of social insurance. It allows a person to pay in for many years at a very low rate in exchange for dependable support in later life, when the risk of illness is higher. Although payments from younger citizens directly fund the Medicare costs of elderly and disabled citizens, the transfer is a mechanism of insurance, not an altruistic effort at redistribution of resources. By making contributions now, young taxpayers gain a right to coverage later. The idea of spreading individual risk over time is another appealing idea of insurance: investing during the prosperous years covers the prospect of calamities later, when income may be limited. This kind of continuity is best achieved by the government, with its ability to track individuals' contributions in the form of taxes, efficiently administered through the Social Security system, and provide access to benefits wherever one happens to be. The government is able to hold together the whole risk pool and guarantee lifelong membership in the plan.

The advantages of government involvement in the business of insurance have not been easy to accept in the United States. Since the 1920s, even private insurance has been branded as socialism by the American Medical Association (AMA) and other physician groups. Still, during the long years of labor unrest in the United States, gradually subdued with the beginning of federal legislation in 1935, employers were at risk and were often the first to appreciate the value of benefit programs to gain loyalty and control employee discontent.[7] Health insurance, sponsored by groups such as the National Civic Federation, became a familiar feature of employee welfare in larger companies.[8] In the United States, private enterprise discovered and developed for-profit insurance. The Depression years actually strengthened private insurance companies. Uncertain times increased the demand for risk management. And when union authority over employee benefit plans was approved in 1947, it represented another major stakeholder in health insurance.

Even with the earliest Blues plans in the 1920s, physicians and hospitals learned to accept insurance as the best way to secure a broad pool of clients with the ability to pay. By 1960, the AMA supported the development of private health insurance, largely to deflect government involvement in health-care financing.[9] By then, private health insurance was an accomplished fact, successfully paying for health care for a large part of the (essentially healthy) working population.

The older adult population, retired from the workforce, presented a new set of challenges. While the working population was increasingly insured, the elderly were generally left out.[10] The elderly have higher rates of illness and disability than the working population, which translate into bad risks from an insurance perspective. Covering the elderly means insuring a group of people who are more likely to claim benefits. Thus, in the private market, older adults face exorbitant premiums or rejection.

This is the context that supported the idea for Medicare. Social insurance is a simple solution to provide universal coverage for a designated population and spread risks over a large pool. The principles of solidarity and security represented in social insurance are explored in detail in chapter 11. The important point here is to recognize the principles of insurance developed in the private market as the model for Medicare financing. The very idea of insurance in government programs has lately come under attack, and it is worth recognizing its foundation in private contract relations—and that it is not a government plot or socialism or un-American at all.

To avoid a monolithic government presence in the everyday operations of health care, Medicare developed a contracting system that allows providers to submit claims to regional intermediaries, once the exclusive preserve of Blue Cross–Blue Shield. Intermediary contracts now involve a wide variety of private insurers. About fifty intermediaries operate across the country, contracting with CMS to process claims for Part A, Part B, home health, and durable medical equipment. For many companies, the Medicare contract provides a major source of income. They in turn play an important role in setting policies defining medical necessity. They are also responsible for educating providers on payment policies and gathering data to pass on to CMS. The intermediaries perform an essentially bureaucratic function. In this arrangement, Medicare mimics the old standard of indemnity insurance, which simply pays out when an eligible claim is submitted. On the other hand, as social insurance, Medicare has a mission to achieve health security, suggesting an open-ended commitment to provide all medically necessary care—one that the program is not equipped to fulfill.

Payment Methods

How we pay for health care creates very clear economic forces. Fee-for-service (FFS) payments to doctors and hospitals have been the dominant model in the United States. Capitation reverses the incentives under FFS: providers have an incentive to keep people out of hospitals and reduce the use of expensive procedures. Instead of overuse, this model can risk the underuse of services. Public trust in HMOs and capitation has been harmed by abuses of "bad" managed care, with profit motives sometimes leading to the denial of urgently needed care.

Good HMOs do exist, however, and they offer many potential advantages for the elderly. If HMOs, in general, are to regain public trust and play a significant role in health care, important issues for the future will be how the monthly rates are set for capitated payments, how much profit is acceptable, and what standards and systems are instituted for quality improvement. All of these issues return to the question of how we pay for care.

Like any system of health insurance, Medicare must decide what benefits to cover and how much to pay providers. The challenge in these decisions is to create a fair system that controls cost, ensures quality, and encourages flexible access to medical care for all beneficiaries. A government agency that concerns itself with these broad issues, as Medicare does, is a groundbreaking achievement. Although set up like a detached indemnity insurer, Medicare has all along operated under a mandate that makes it the natural ally of those promoting improvement and reform in health care.

FEE-FOR-SERVICE

When Medicare was enacted, providers were paid on an FFS basis. Hospitals, nursing homes, home health-care providers, and physicians were reimbursed for any covered service received by a patient. Originally, the fee was set slightly above estimated "reasonable" costs. Analysts generally agree that this reimbursement system contributed significantly to the rapid increases in health care costs in the 1970s and early 1980s. Because FFS rewards providers for doing more, it creates incentives for "overuse"—offering unnecessary services and tests.

Hospital costs escalated rapidly in Medicare's first two decades. Prices for each service and treatment were contained, but the open-ended reimbursement encouraged more intensive treatments and tests and a proliferation of services.[11] For physicians, charges were supposed to be "customary," set at a rate accepted by a majority of physicians in the community. Without an official, standardized physician fee schedule, however, this definition was elusive, and physicians could easily raise their fees. Moreover, new technology and experimental treatments that were at first time-consuming and expensive stayed expensive even after they had become routine and easier to perform because the system offered no incentive for physicians to lower prices.

Medicare was not the only insurer facing rapidly rising costs, but it began to shoulder a larger share of the burden. Between 1967 and 1983, total private expenditures for hospital services grew an average of 13.9 percent per year; Medicare's grew 17.3 percent. Private expenditures for physician services grew an average of 12.4 percent per year; Medicare's grew 16.4 percent.[12] Growth in hospital costs slowed noticeably once prospective payment with diagnosis-related groups (DRGs) was introduced in 1983 (see below). From 1980 to 1989, the average real growth in Medicare expenditures per beneficiary slowed to 3.5 percent for Part A, compared to 8.2 percent for Part B.[13]

Physicians' fees, which had continued to rise rapidly, were finally brought under some control in 1992, when Medicare established a fee schedule that set limits in advance. In this process, the legacy of Medicare politics that had been hashed out thirty years before to favor providers reemerged. The AMA lobbied strenuously against the government's right to impose a fee schedule, even though the practice was by then already common among commercial insurance companies.

In the 1970s, medical ethics supported the idea that it was not a physician's responsibility to worry about how much a procedure cost or whether a less expensive procedure or test might be almost as effective for the patient. The physician was seen as the advocate for the individual patient, not for a health plan or the national Medicare budget. Respected experts encouraged physicians to tend to their patients and "let society decide" how to set limits on escalating costs. In a seminal essay in the *New England Journal of Medicine,* Howard Hiatt wrote, "It is surely not fair to ask the physician or other medical care provider to set [national health priorities] in the context of his or her own medical practice."[14] Instead, he argued, society as a whole must determine its health priorities and then educate physicians on how to adhere to them. One could argue that the Medicare program was a vehicle for society to decide how much it wanted to pay for health care.

By 1980, advancing costs were colliding with a major obstacle: payers. Businesses buying employee benefits, insurance carriers, and federal and state government agencies buying services for Medicaid, Medicare, and other groups all began to feel the squeeze. This collision became a factor in health-insurance debates that had been simmering for decades among politicians, physicians, and insurance companies. By ensuring a payment mechanism for hospitals and health-care providers, Medicare had created a steady market for scientific and technological advances in medicine but was unwilling to cover everything that might be medically necessary, like medications, and many preventive services. Patients were left with unsettling gaps in coverage that discouraged the best coordination of services. These gaps are becoming increasingly expensive for those who need care.

PROSPECTIVE PAYMENT

In the 1980s, Congress began to try to control rising Medicare costs. First instituted in 1983, the hospital prospective payment system (PPS) reimburses hospitals, nursing homes, and home health-care agencies on the basis of diagnosis-related groups. For each defined medical condition, a set payment is established that represents the average cost of an episode of care for patients with this diagnosis. For example, a hospital is paid a set amount to care for an episode of pneumonia, even if one case requires more expensive services or a longer hospital stay. Initially, hospitals received the same payment for treating two Medicare patients with pneumonia, even if one was sixty-five years old and the other ninety-five and suffering from other chronic conditions. To protect hospitals from large financial losses due to unusually expensive cases, adjustments in the late 1980s made allowances for older or sicker patients, and "outlier" payments were offered for extremely long hospitalizations resulting from complications.

When a hospital submits a claim for a Medicare patient to its fiscal intermediary or carrier, the bill shows a principal diagnosis, along with other information that allows the intermediary to determine the applicable DRG. The DRG amount constitutes payment in full for the patient's treatment, regardless of the actual services rendered. Numerous variations are possible. Payments to hospitals are based on the standard DRG amount, plus add-ons for certain hospital and patient characteristics. Add-ons account for regional wage differentials; case mix (to compensate hospitals serving a "disproportionate share" of low-income patients); designation as a teaching hospital; and outliers, covering anomalous cases with unusually high costs.[15]

Prospective payment is intended to create an incentive to reduce unnecessary costs. The implementation of prospective payment by Medicare shook the hospital industry in the 1980s and brought a new budget consciousness to hospital administrators. Pressure mounted to reduce the length of hospital stays and to discharge patients earlier. This incentive has improved efficiency tremendously in some areas, like the increasing use of day surgery, but may also result in discharging patients who are not yet fully recovered. Readmission soon after discharge has become an indicator that the patient was discharged too soon.

Early discharge can also put a heavy burden on families. Patients sometimes say they have been pushed out of the hospital because "the DRG ran out." Such statements reveal a misunderstanding about how DRGs work. Medicare does not set a limit on how long a patient may stay in the hospital. The DRG for a given condition is an estimate of *average* cost, so some cases will cost more and others less; but costs should balance out if the hospital has a mix of patients. If complications cause an extremely long hospitalization, Medicare will pay an extra "outlier" rate. The DRG system is not intended to encourage hospitals to discharge patients before they are ready to leave, only to avoid unnecessarily long hospital stays.

For the most part, Medicare's DRG system has been judged successful at reducing costs.[16] Studies suggest that some hospital costs have been transferred to skilled-nursing facilities (SNFs) or nursing homes and home health-care providers, for which Medicare reimburses a small fraction of the costs separately from the hospital DRG. Under this system, a number of hospitals have been able to maximize payment for rehabilitative care by designating a number of beds as a skilled-nursing unit; they can thereby access another fund of Medicare dollars for the same patient. Home health and SNF costs increased rapidly in the 1990s. The diversification of care probably represents more efficient teamwork in many cases, but too often it borders on unloading expensive cases to avoid the hospital cost. This incentive was blocked by reforms in 1997 that created another system of prospective payment for skilled nursing, called resource utilization groups (RUGs), patterned on DRGs. The new system has made nursing homes more vigilant about accepting inappropriate transfers from the hospital.

A system based on reimbursing for "average" costs of care makes it more difficult to cover care for the small percentage of individuals with the most expensive needs.[17] One way to remedy the problem is to adjust payments upward for more severe cases. The additional DRG weights for "outliers" are one example of Medicare's innovation in this area. Nonetheless, providers continue to face uncertainties and risk; at the same time, a vigorous patients' rights movement has developed in response to perceptions that hospitals are cutting corners under prospective payment.

In spite of genuine problems with selection bias and denial of care, it should be emphasized that the simple existence of profit does not necessarily indicate wrongdoing. Prospective payment transfers risk to the providers of care, and they accept that risk with the promise that efficiency and risk will be rewarded and that they will be paid enough at least to cover their operating and capital costs. Profit for assuming risk is to be expected and may be used to cover less profitable services. Yet CMS closely monitors profit margins on its DRG codes and regularly restricts payments. Studies are conducted by the inspector general of the Department of Health and Human Services and other contracted researchers, who are worried about the effects of reduced profit margins on access and quality. Many hospital SNF units could not survive and closed once the RUG system was enacted. Although Medicare's system of prospective payment appears to be working to control costs, it puts providers in the awkward position of accepting a dictated price as well as a financial risk borne without compensation. Today there is a general retreat from capitation as a payment model in the private market, but it continues to work well for certain experienced, well-organized, and largely nonprofit delivery systems.[18]

Medicare's system of prospective payment tends to set one sector of the health care system against another, particularly as it pays very little for long-term care or rehabilitation. Hospitals discharge patients to maximize income, and nursing homes shoulder the burden. Some larger incentive is needed to integrate acute and subacute aspects of care, allowing people to recover outside the hospital or avoid hospitalization altogether.

Demonstration projects promoting coordinated community care for the elderly are proceeding in the United States and in several other countries, mostly using prospective payment schemes. (PACE programs in the U.S. are addressed in chapter 4.) In general, they show that geriatric assessment and intensive case management, combined with flexible treatment options and facilities, do produce better health outcomes and quality of life and may save money.[19]

HMOS FOLLOW THE MONEY

Different approaches to managed care developed in the 1980s in an effort to control the unsustainable inflation in health-care costs. HMOs exist in three main forms, with some variations. Managed care organizations (MCOs) represent systems that combine finance and health-care delivery. Preferred-provider organizations (PPOs) represent agencies that develop and sell the services of broad provider networks (usually physician-dominated). Provider-sponsored organizations (PSOs) represent providers capable of bearing risk and providing a full range of services; they deal directly with purchasers, without an insurance carrier or other intermediary.

One new direction was based on a few notable and longstanding examples of nonprofit HMOs, like Kaiser Permanente (established in the 1950s) and the Harvard Community Health Plan (created in the 1960s). The idea of "health maintenance" derived from the premise that capitation (as opposed to FFS) created both an incentive and the flexibility to invest in keeping people healthy rather than treating them only after they become ill. In the first proud years of managed care, HMOs claimed a new understanding of cost-effectiveness, both controlling prices and improving the quality of patient care. Also, by the 1980s physicians began to accept some responsibility for avoiding unnecessary expenses without compromising care.

One of the innovations of these organizations was to train medical interns and residents about the costs of tests, treatments, and medications. Physicians performed fewer expensive tests and services when they were regularly informed of the costs. Costs rose to normal, however, once the physicians stopped receiving regular updates on cost increases.[20] This finding supports the reputation of HMOs as information experts and data warehouses. The best health systems provide feedback on patient outcomes as well as on costs. With intensive information campaigns, responsible HMOs are able to satisfy government regulatory agencies and also direct their efficiency and quality programs at the point of service to encourage more effective practices. Innovative HMOs paid physicians a flat salary; and in some cases, they shared risks with the HMO through capitated payments in order to curb the expensive and wasteful use of unnecessary services that prevailed under FFS.

In 1997, because of the good track record of the HMO model and the obvious advantages of prospective payment, Congress expanded the availability of managed care to Medicare beneficiaries with its Medicare+Choice program. M+C allowed monthly fees to HMOs who agreed to cover a defined set of services to Medicare patients—like an HMO.

Many insurance companies and provider systems entered the new market for M+C contracts, with the promise that efficient use of services could lead to profit margins. Growing throughout the 1990s, enrollment of Medicare beneficiaries in various types of contracted managed care peaked in 1999 at 6.3 million, or 16 percent of the noninstitutionalized Medicare population. The experience for many insurance carriers was disillusioning. New companies began to leave the market, and established companies began to withdraw from less profitable areas on a county-by-county basis. By 2001, the number of Medicare beneficiaries enrolled in M+C plans had fallen to 5.6 million (14 percent), and by 2003 to 4.6 million (12 percent).[21] Many of the companies were ill-equipped to manage care for the elderly population. Those that have been successful have large systems of care and considerable expertise in geriatric medical teams.

Marketing strategies emphasizing the unproven assertion that wide choice of doctors leads to higher quality care have reduced consumer interest in traditional HMOs and led to the growth of the loose affiliations of doctors in PPOs. PPOs are now the predominant form of organization for financing health-care delivery. It remains uncertain whether these organizations possess either the capacity or motivation to measure performance and control costs.[22] PPOs are often large national or regional organizations that rely on the scope of their networks and discounted fees to appeal to health-care purchasers, but they do not have an organized system of care delivery. Unlike HMOs, a PPO bears no financial risk in its contracts but charges a network access fee and processes claims for the purchaser. The purchaser is usually a self-insured employee benefit plan or other fully insured payer, which bears the risk of providing health insurance.[23] PPOs tailor their activities to their clients and may implement utilization management (screening to reduce unnecessary services) or prescription-drug formularies on request, but, like Medicare intermediaries and insurance companies, they are really only set up to process claims data.

Fee-for-service reimbursement persists in most of American medicine, reinforcing the idea that more is better. As Alain Enthoven points out, this arrangement was fine when medicine was limited in what it could do, choice was limited, and costs were a fraction of what they are today.[24] Before 1970, efficiency in the financing and delivery of health care was not much of an issue. Today we can do more, and we expect more. Yet, in spite of all efforts, costs are still spiraling out of control.

PHYSICIAN PAYMENT REFORM

Another attempt to control the rising costs of Medicare came in 1992 with a new fee schedule for physician payments. Medicare originally paid physicians by fees determined to be "customary, prevailing, and reasonable" (CPR). The policy was adopted to gain the AMA's initial cooperation with Medicare.[25] By the late 1980s, expenditures for Medicare physician services were increasing at a faster rate than Medicare hospital expenditures and overall national health-care expenditures, and they far outpaced the rate of inflation. By 1990, Medicare cost taxpayers $100 billion per year, the largest domestic public program after Social Security, and Part B spending on physician care represented 40 percent of total Medicare costs. Even adjusted for inflation, Medicare physician payments per beneficiary more than doubled during the 1980s. This situation resulted partly from hospital DRGs, which created an incentive to perform many services in outpatient settings. And new technology made outpatient treatments more feasible.

Physician payments were not only demanding a larger share of the budget but also were responsible for serious distortions and disparities in physicians' incomes, particularly between primary care and surgical specialties and between physicians in different geographic regions. Under the CPR system, Medicare tended to pay much more for technical procedures and much less for diagnosis by office visits, patient history, and physical examination. This is one reason why young physicians today are less attracted to careers in primary care or geriatric medicine, where time is spent in communication, patient education, and complex chronic-care management. Recently, Medicare recognized this aspect of care with a new payment category called "evaluation and management," which does not solve the problem of unbalanced compensation but at least addresses it and opens a new avenue for negotiation.

Recognizing that the customary fees were not the result of real market forces, policy makers began to realize the importance of creating a more equitable payment scale.[26] Physicians, too, were becoming disillusioned with the administrative burdens of the CPR system. Signs of collapse were appearing. In 1984 Congress froze Medicare fee increases and two years later restricted balance billing—the amount physicians can charge patients above the Medicare-approved rate. After experience with the prospective-payment system for hospital services demonstrated that reimbursement reform could contain health-care costs, Congress was encouraged to tackle the problem of physician fees with a similar solution.

Congress had already created the Physician Payment Review Commission (PPRC) in 1985 to study options and make recommendations for a reasonable, workable payment plan for physicians. The PPRC later merged with the Prospective Payment Assessment Commission (ProPAC), which advised Congress on hospital payments. The combined organization exists now as the Medicare Payment Advisory Committee (MedPAC).

PPRC played a unique role in enacting physician payment reform. In 1988, Congress directed the commission to recommend ways to control Medicare expenditures for physician services. There were several hurdles. First, the medical lobby, especially the AMA, needed to be convinced that a fee schedule would not threaten professional autonomy or physicians' incomes in general. The commission also had to overcome the argument of free-market advocates that fee schedules in general constitute unwarranted government intrusions into the marketplace. (Interestingly, while the AMA had opposed Medicare in 1965, by 1985 the medical lobby was working to keep Medicare rates high, an effort inconsistent with free-market principles.)

The absence of traditional market forces in health care generally, and in Medicare coverage particularly, makes it easier to justify a fee schedule (and public resistance to tax increases makes it unavoidable). However, this lack of traditional market forces also meant that PPRC had to establish a rational relationship between price and quality, and this task was the committee's greatest challenge. Medicare has to pay rates close enough to market prices to ensure that providers will continue to treat patients, especially in underserved areas where access is threatened.

Given these conditions, Congress asked a group of Harvard researchers, led by William Hsiao, to create a physician fee schedule that would manage to capture value and provide fair compensation for providers of relatively similar care. The result was a system matching price to costs called the resource-based relative-value scale (RBRVS), which uses a formula to base payments for physician work on the resources used.

At this time the principles of care management, linked with primary care and geriatric medicine, were beginning to be recognized. Both fields can reduce unnecessary hospital use, tests, and treatments. Yet specialists are paid so little in these fields that it has been hard to convince young doctors to train for them and hard to retain specialists who have done so. One hope was that RBRVS could right this imbalance and adjust payments across specialties to encourage the most efficient medical care.

PPRC reviewed Hsiao's recommendations, made some modifications, and then forwarded the RBRVS system to Congress. As it turned out, the playing field was not leveled. High-tech specialists lobbied to protect their payment rates; and, because Medicare has always been a political target sensitive to the demands of interest groups, these highly paid specialists became disproportionately influential in the fee-setting process.

PPRC also considered other alternatives: a refined CPR system, prospective payment similar to DRGs, and capitation. The fee schedule was chosen as the least radical solution. The commission made it clear, however, that other solutions might be recommended at a later time if the fee schedule proved ineffective in reducing Medicare physician payments. Interestingly, the talk of prepayment capitation and DRGs helped PPRC gain the support of the AMA and other physician groups: the new fee schedule was viewed as preferable. Because surgical fees were expected to decrease and primary care fees to increase under the fee schedule, surgeons and other procedure-oriented specialists opposed it, and primary-care specialists supported it.

Beneficiaries at first worried that the fee schedule would result in increased out-of-pocket costs if physicians decided to make up for lower Medicare reimbursements by billing patients directly. PPRC addressed these concerns by recommending restrictions on "balance billing" by physicians. A "participating provider" program was introduced in 1984 to encourage physicians to accept "assignment."[27] Participants receive higher payments and more timely processing in exchange for assuring access for beneficiaries and accepting the assigned fee as payment in full.[28] Participation rates vary by specialty, from about one-third to three-fourths of physicians in any particular group in 1992; the overall rate increased to about 80 percent of all physicians by 1997. In 2004, MedPAC found that 88 percent of beneficiaries reported little or no trouble finding a primary care physician, and 94 percent had no problem locating a specialist who accepted Medicare.[29]

The reform succeeded because researchers, politicians, and varied interest groups were able to work together to devise a compromise plan they could all live with, even though no group thought it ideal. Throughout the process, PPRC played an important and unique advisory role. As an arm of Congress, the commission was free of any obligations to the executive branch, and members of Congress were therefore more willing to trust its analysis. Negotiations were coordinated in public, with discussion and participation from all parties solicited; and this open debate succeeded in spite of the complex issues and interests intrinsic to all Medicare policy. Today, the PPRC successor commission, MedPAC, is at the forefront of all discussion on Medicare payment reform.

The Choppy Sea of Fee Schedules

In some important ways, RBRVS has not fulfilled its promise. The fee schedule has slowed the growth of Medicare payments to physicians, but the rate of growth remains well above the rate of inflation.[30] More importantly, physicians have an incentive to increase the volume of procedures they perform and the number of patients they see to maintain their salary levels. This kind of behavior, called physician-induced demand, is a characteristic of many FFS systems. RBRVS did not manage to change physician practice patterns.

To understand the inequities of the physician fee schedule, consider the following scenario.

Mrs. Margaret Lofton, a seventy-five-year-old woman, finds a lump in her breast during a breast self-examination in the shower. Panicked and sure she is going to die, she calls her daughter, who brings her to her primary physician, a geriatrician at a large hospital in New York. The geriatrician tells Mrs. Lofton not to worry. She just needs to get a mammogram to see if the lump is cancerous. Even if it is, breast cancer is usually not as aggressive in women of her age as it is in younger women. Sensing her anxiety, the physician asks her to describe what is worrying her most about her possible illness. Mrs. Lofton finally tells the physician that she is anxious because she lives alone and does not want her daughter to have to miss work to be with her. Her physician takes the time to talk to her about possible options, such as home care, and refers her to a social worker in her community who specializes in senior issues. The referral gives Mrs. Lofton someone to talk to about her anxiety and also someone who can coordinate services if it becomes necessary.

Mrs. Lofton then goes to the radiologist for a mammogram. A biopsy shows the lump is cancerous. She returns to the radiologist for a bone scan and an MRI to find out whether the cancer has spread. Luckily, it seems her cancer is contained locally. Her treatment options are a lumpectomy or a mastectomy. After several long talks with her geriatrician, she opts for a mastectomy because it requires less follow-up radiation treatment: she does not want to make the trip to the radiation office as frequently as she would need with a lumpectomy, and she certainly does not want her daughter to take time off work each day to shuttle her to the clinic.

A surgeon performs Mrs. Lofton's mastectomy. Two days later, she goes home under the supervision of her geriatrician, who makes sure her blood pressure and diabetes are controlled after surgery. Mrs. Lofton is delirious and unsteady when she first comes home. During a home visit, the geriatrician determines that these symptoms are due to a new sleeping medication and two other drugs that should have been stopped when she left the hospital.

Mrs. Lofton's daughter takes some time off work to care for her. Mrs. Lofton also qualifies for a home health nurse to come to her home to help several hours a day. The social worker signs her up for Meals on Wheels, and she receives a hot lunch every day. She needs continuing treatment for hypertension, chronic thyroid disease, arthritis, and irritable bowel disease, all provided by her geriatrician. Her daughter is now concerned about her own risk for cancer, since she is taking an estrogen replacement to reduce the symptoms of menopause and prevent osteoporosis. The geriatrician talks with her at length about her concerns and refers the daughter to a women's health program for follow-up and counseling. A year later, Mrs. Lofton continues to see her geriatrician and oncologist for checkups; she feels things are pretty much back to normal in her life.

This patient and her daughter are lucky. She had a geriatrician willing to coordinate her care, answer her questions, and listen to her concerns. She received the care she needed for her cancer. And she got the help she needed at home as well. How much did each of Mrs. Lofton's physicians get paid for the services they provided? (CPT is the payment code.)

Diagnostic mammogram (CPT 76091, bilateral mammogram): $119

Mastectomy (CPT Code 19200): $1,300

Office visits with geriatrician, depending on length and nature of the visit (CPT 99241–99244): $13 to $143[31]

The mammogram charge is for the physician's professional services, with an additional payment for use of the equipment. Technicians paid by the hospital perform the procedure, and the physician spends a few minutes reading the mammogram. The radiologist is paid up to one hundred times more than the geriatrician for the same amount of time. Comparing the mastectomy with the longer office visits, the time actually spent with the patient is about the same, yet the surgeon is paid ten times as much as the geriatrician. To make matters more difficult, the physician in an office gets no additional Medicare support for the staffing there, while Part A hospital payments provide all the staff support for the more highly paid hospital-based specialists. The office geriatrician has to pay the nurses himself, while the hospital surgeon or radiologist does not.

Discrepancies like this have led to extensive analysis and debate in the medical community. Do such differences in billing between counseling services and technical procedures make market sense? Surgical skills take a long time to develop and thus probably should be compensated at a higher rate—but how much higher? Without conscientious coordination of her care, Mrs. Lofton might have fallen through the cracks, developed complications from medication interactions or diabetes or both, failed to get her breast cancer diagnosed or treated until it was too late, or failed to get the help she needed when she arrived home after her surgery. These questions of value are not resolved by the invisible hand of market forces, but rather in a fee structure determined by Medicare.

Negotiating Values

Although there is a formal process for changing the physician fee schedule, the law requires budget neutrality, meaning that total physician payments must remain constant. This places the medical profession in a zero-sum game: if payments for one group, such as geriatricians, are to increase, some other specialty will lose revenue.

RVS UPDATE COMMITTEE (RUC)

Annual updates to the relative-value units (RVUs) are based on recommendations from a committee called the AMA/Specialty RVS Update Committee (RUC), which includes representatives from both the AMA and various medical-specialty societies. RUC was formed in 1991 to convince the AMA to endorse the fee schedule.[32] The committee makes annual recommendations to CMS on the fee schedule.

The committee is composed of twenty-nine members. Six seats are reserved for representatives of the AMA, the Osteopathic Association, the CPT Editorial Panel, the Health Care Professionals Advisory Committee, the Practice Expense Advisory Committee, and a chair appointed by the AMA. The remaining twenty-three seats are reserved for representatives from major medical specialties. Family medicine and pediatrics are assigned one seat each. Three seats rotate every two years, two for subspecialties in internal medicine and one for any other specialty not already represented. On the current roster, geriatric medicine happens to be one of the rotating seats. Thus the payment-review committee for Medicare, a program for the elderly, assigns geriatric medicine one seat among twenty-nine, and only for two years in every ten or twenty. Clearly, geriatric medicine has little power or influence over Medicare payment policies, even though older adults are ultimately the major point of interest in all the deliberations.

RUC membership shows a preponderance of highly paid specialist groups. Since RUC is bound by budget neutrality, those physicians representing specialties that benefit from the current fee schedule have no incentive to recommend major payment increases for other, lower-paid services.

Listening and talking to patients and families is a time-consuming and important part of practicing medicine. Time spent with the physician is often the experience most highly valued by patients and most often missed in modern health care. CPT quirks include a dermatologist's being paid $200 for three minutes removing a malignant skin lesion in the office, with additional payment for each biopsy of the removed lesion, while a geriatrician is paid $100 for a thirty-minute patient-and-family visit to evaluate mental confusion. In the same thirty minutes, the dermatologist could earn $2,000 doing ten biopsies.

The current fee schedule creates a "technology imperative" that encourages physicians to spend less time talking to patients and more time performing technical procedures, some of which are of marginal significance or not clearly necessary. Although the RBRVS system has successfully imposed a degree of economy on physician reimbursement, the persistence of the technology imperative shows that it has done little to change the incentives embedded in the fee-for-service system. The AMA publishes lists of those CPT codes that make up the largest percentage of incomes by specialty. All of the fees have been reduced by RBRVS, making it all the more unlikely that specialists on the RUC would support a reallocation to favor geriatrics.

Fee discrepancies between the most commonly performed activities of internists and surgeons are reflected in income differences. The AMA reports the median 1997 income for physicians in primary care at $140,000, compared to $195,000 for other specialists.[33] Other estimates show more dramatic differences. According to the *Physician Compensation and Production Survey* of the Medical Group Management Association (MGMA), the 1998 median income of physicians in internal medicine was $141,147, compared to $271,828 for diagnostic radiologists and $455,574 for cardiovascular surgeons, the highest-paid specialty on the list.[34] Such averages mask a much greater range of values for individual income levels. Disparities are exaggerated because hospitals are paid more for the high technology treatments and thus are more willing to support the higher earning specialists with staff and facilities.

In 1988, before RBRVS was implemented, Hsiao and colleagues published an article in the *New England Journal of Medicine* describing the system and its potential benefits, referring in part to the unfair payment discrepancies between primary care and high-tech procedures: "Roughly speaking, evaluation-and-management services are currently compensated at less than half the rate of invasive services."[35] Such payment discrepancies are at least as dramatic today. Young physicians have little financial incentive to enter specialties such as geriatrics that require more lengthy consultations and fewer procedures. Primary-care generalists in internal medicine and family practice do better by seeing more younger patients who have less complex problems. The current shortage of geriatric-oriented specialists will be felt more severely once the boomers come of age.

MEDICARE FRAUD

Some policy makers focus on fraud as a major problem in Medicare. While safeguards are needed to avoid real abuses, sometimes these regulations can restrict the flexibility needed for good geriatric care. Geriatric care requires medical services that are flexible and geared to individual needs, not hard-and-fast disease categories. How to achieve this flexibility in a fee-for-service world is not abundantly clear. Appropriate oversight and quality-control mechanisms need to be part of the system to reduce opportunities for fraud and abuse, but such mechanisms must also avoid stifling quality care.

Medical necessity is the model used by Medicare and other insurers to determine what they will pay for, but the term may be defined differently in practice by a geriatrician, physical therapist, and surgeon. In addition to managing potential disagreements over what constitutes a legitimate claim for payment, providers must also navigate both state and federal laws prohibiting self-referral, protections for patient safety and rights, restrictions on marketing practices, monitoring investments, and many other complex regulations.

One example of a disputed service is physical therapy, which was initially only covered for patients recovering from an acute illness, such as a stroke. As soon as improvement tailed off, coverage was discontinued. Now Medicare recognizes that for very frail elders, maintenance of function is critically important. Being able to go to the bathroom unaided can mean the difference between living independently and moving to a nursing home, and a weak older patient may need ongoing therapy to maintain that function. Physical activity can prevent exacerbations of medical conditions such as vascular insufficiency, diabetes, pneumonia, and even depression. Even though Medicare has loosened its requirement for documented improvement from physical therapy, some fiscal intermediaries are more rigid than others in how they interpret medical necessity; and there are numerous cases where decisions have been appealed. Ambiguity in such cases makes physicians likely to err on the side of undertreatment to avoid any possibility of a fraud investigation. Even knowing you are acting in the patient's interests does not counteract the chilling effect of facing a potential federal investigation.[36]

Only a small number of unethical providers knowingly defraud Medicare. Many more may be disposed to stretch the truth to be sure a needed service is provided to a patient.[37] Some argue that more flexible and reasonable Medicare rules and payment systems would diminish the temptation to "fudge the rules," but such assertions ignore the value of having a standard by which payment disparities can be measured and enforced. No one expects the stock market or corporate finance, for example, to run honestly without the supervision of the Securities and Exchange Commission (and not even then). Similarly, the large sums of money involved in the health-care industry create big incentives for fraud. In consequence laws have been developed to protect the taxpayers' dollars.

Although many providers who participate in Medicare voice legitimate concerns that Medicare rules sometimes prevent them from providing the best care, CMS has voiced equally legitimate concerns that the agency is responsible for preventing Medicare dollars from being spent on unnecessary or nonexistent services. This is just the kind of behavior a market expects from a prudent purchaser. CMS is responsible for spending billions of taxpayer dollars efficiently and in the best interest of beneficiaries. The controversial point here may simply be that contracting with the government requires greater rectitude than with any other customer. Normally, a dissatisfied customer may simply not come back, but the government is likely to come back—in force.[38] Overreaching enforcement leads to reports of raids, harsh fines, and incarceration. Maintaining the public trust requires a wide range of available enforcement options that promote cost-effective treatment but do not discourage medical professionals from performing valuable services.

Although a valid concern, efforts to educate consumers have resulted in a misperception that fraud and abuse are widespread. Polls show that about 70 percent of citizens across all age groups think fraud and abuse are major reasons why Medicare faces financial difficulties. About 20 percent think eliminating fraud and abuse from Medicare would be enough to assure the program's solvency.[39] Clearly, too much emphasis on fraud and abuse diverts public attention from Medicare's broader, more systemic problems, which cost considerably more, both in financing and health outcomes. Even if no fraud and abuse existed in Medicare, paying the health-care costs of the baby boomers while ensuring quality care is going to present an enormous national challenge.

Payment Challenges

Mrs. Lofton's story focused on payment disparities for physicians but left out the important details of her own out-of-pocket expenses. The burden on patients, in the forms of increasing amounts for deductibles and co-payments and rising outpatient drug costs, is a central theme in Medicare finances. Mrs. Lofton's medication might cost her more than $1000 per month. Her medication costs are at a level not eligible for reimbursement from the new Medicare drug benefits. A Medigap policy to cover some of these costs would itself incur a monthly premium that might cost several hundred dollars. Such policies are often subject to experience rating, meaning higher costs for those like Mrs. Lofton who need the coverage most.

In addition to Mrs. Lofton's own expenses, her daughter lost income by missing several weeks of work. Such direct costs to family members are often neglected in out-of-pocket expense calculations. Although Mrs.

Lofton and her family were able to navigate to a successful outcome despite the gaps in her Medicare coverage, other families find the gaps more difficult to manage.

Insurance is both a way of spreading risk and of paying for services. Any insurance plan faces the complex challenge of establishing fair rates—not so high that Medicare costs are unsustainable and not so low that services are not available. Payment policies often seem irrational and highly political—subject to pressures from providers who want more money, interest groups that oppose government programs on principle, and taxpayers who resist higher tax bills. In this environment, it is easy to see the barriers to changes that would pay for good geriatric medicine, coordination of care, and evidence-based limits on spending. Instead, we now expect patients to be better informed consumers and to pay more of the cost themselves.

CHAPTER 9

Prescription Drugs

The Challenge Remains

Today, no one would consider creating a health-insurance program for elders without including coverage for medications. When the Medicare law was drafted in 1965, coverage of prescription drugs was discussed briefly, but the issue was dropped as part of a compromise. Drugs were not used as widely in 1965 as they are today and were not considered a catastrophic expense. Since then, a steady stream of new medications has helped to improve the quality of life for many people, but they have come at a price. Today, prescription drugs are the fastest-growing category of personal health expenditures. Commercial insurers have begun covering prescription drugs, but Medicare has been reluctant to absorb the enormous new costs. Powerful interests squared off in the creation of a drug benefit for the Medicare Prescription Drug Improvement and Modernization Act of 2003 (MMA), creating a benefit that promises to be both expensive and ineffective. It seems likely that the controversy over how best to provide this coverage will continue in the next few years.

Industry Growth

Before the 1990s, the growth in hospital and physician services eclipsed expenditures for prescription drugs, reducing the pharmaceutical share of total health-care expenditures to less than 6 percent. A surge of expansion since 1995 has increased this to more than 10 percent, with annual growth rates rising from 6.5 percent in 1993 to 26 percent in 1999.[1] Even as growth in other sectors of the health-care market has moderated in recent years, expenditures for drugs have continued to escalate.

Pharmaceutical companies generate controversy because of their colossal marketing budgets and profit margins, about four times higher than the average for all Fortune 500 firms. For the major pharmaceutical manufacturers, marketing takes up 34 percent of total operating expenses; only 14 percent is devoted to research and development. The bulk of drug marketing concentrates on "detailing" for physicians, who are given free samples to encourage them to prescribe the company's drugs. After 1997, when the U.S. Food and Drug Administration (FDA) relaxed the rules on drug advertising, direct-to-consumer advertising rapidly increased, taking up about $2.5 billion of a $15.7 billion marketing budget for the industry by 2000.[2]

Criticism of high drug prices is accompanied by ready acknowledgment that new medications improve medical effectiveness.[3] Outpatient treatment of diseases with a drug regimen and close medical monitoring can replace hospitalization, surgeries, and other expensive, invasive, uncomfortable, or risky procedures. The appropriate use of prescription drugs can actually reduce total treatment costs. In some cases, drugs are the only effective treatment available. But appropriate treatment isn't always the newest or most expensive drug, especially for the elderly.

The costs of drug expenditures for private insurers rose from almost nothing in 1965 to about one-third of total costs in 1990 and over half by 1998.[4] During the same period, patients went from paying almost all drug costs directly to paying only one-fourth by 1998.[5] Nevertheless, patients' out-of-pocket costs have increased.[6] For the elderly Medicare population, the trend is reflected in recent and projected changes in employer-based insurance policies, which are shifting more costs to retirees.[7] It is likely that even with the new MMA coverage, out-of-pocket expenses will grow. Similarly, Medigap supplemental policies that cover drugs increased their premiums by over one-third between 1998 and 2000. Trends in Medicare managed care are the same.[8]

Although prescription drugs account for only 10 percent of all personal health-care expenditures, compared to 36 percent for hospital care and 25 percent for physician and clinical services, national spending on drugs is increasing two to five times faster than spending on hospital or physician services.[9] On average, total prescription drug spending increased about 13 percent each year between 1993 and 2000, with projections of about 12 percent through the next decade. Nearly half (48 percent) of the increasing costs for prescription drugs through the 1990s are attributable to greater use of prescription drugs, both because they are being used more and because they are more costly.[10] Price increases accounted for about one-fourth of the rise in spending on prescription drugs from 1997 to 2000. Between 1998 and 2000, prescription drug prices rose at more than three times the rate of inflation. The remaining 28 percent of rising costs was due to the type of prescription, indicating a shift from older drugs to newer, more expensive drugs.

Direct-to-Consumer Advertising

Heavy investment in advertising to fuel demand for prescription drugs is a controversial issue, even though in other areas of the economy advertising is usually perceived as a good way to promote product awareness and sales. Physicians worry about advertising undermining their professional authority and creating demand for potentially risky or unnecessary medications.[11] Since Food and Drug Administration (FDA) regulations were eased in 1997, drugs have been advertised widely on television, where commercials encourage patients to ask their physicians about the featured drug.

In some situations, advertising can educate and empower the consumer. Ads may prompt people to recognize a medical problem and seek necessary treatment. A serious drawback, however, is that ads do not discuss the evidence supporting use of a particular drug or, more important, provide information about the illness it is intended to treat. Taking the right drug can save one's life. Taking the wrong drug can be a dangerous and costly mistake, and not only to the patient. In a 1999 tort case concerning the directly advertised contraceptive Norplant, the New Jersey Supreme Court held the manufacturer, and not physicians, liable for the injuries sustained.[12] The decision indicates a new area of uncertainty about who is responsible for adequately warning about the risks of medications that are advertised directly to consumers. Recent disclosures of adverse effects of Vioxx and similar pain treatments will lead to more big legal challenges for the industry.

Nonetheless, direct advertising works. In 1999, for instance, when Schering-Plough spent $137 million advertising its allergy drug Claritin, sales rose 21 percent. When AstraZeneca spent $79.4 million to advertise Prilosec, a drug used to treat ulcers, sales rose 24 percent. When Bristol Myers Squibb spent $43 million to advertise Glucophage, an oral diabetes drug, sales rose about 50 percent.[13] The sales increases did not reflect any scientific evidence that these were the best treatments in their class.

Ideally, patients and physicians would be able to obtain information about the least expensive drug for a particular condition. Unfortunately, reliable clinical comparisons of effectiveness matched to price are rare, so clinical decisions are usually made without taking price into account. In many cases, the bulk of the price is charged to an insurer anyway, so there is little incentive for the consumer to limit costs. As for the physician, research confirms that physicians tend to underestimate prices for expensive drugs and overestimate prices for inexpensive ones.[14] Physicians indicate a willingness to consider price if the information were easily and reliably available.[15]

In all areas of health care, there is a professional movement towards evidence-based medicine—the idea that medical decisions should be based on systematically examined scientific evidence about what works best. The idea of making medical decisions based on evidence seems obvious, but the volume of new research is too overwhelming for any individual to master. Physicians also tend to be conservative in their prescribing habits, preferring to stick with drugs they know about (or that the friendly drug company rep has briefed them about), regardless of price, and they don't have the time or resources to research all possible alternatives. There are, however, good alternatives. For example, formulary systems that recommend preferred drugs, and reference pricing that identifies the least expensive effective drug in a class, would enable Medicare to cover more drug costs and encourage use of the safest and most effective medications. These techniques are used in large, high-quality health systems, but both are explicitly forbidden in the recent MMA law.

The competing values of evidence-based medicine and drug advertising highlight a key issue in health-care reform. The goal of advertising is to sell; the goal of medicine is to heal, using the most appropriate products regardless of brand name or advertising efforts. Health care does not conform well to market principles, and the result of intensive drug advertising may be unnecessarily high costs or poor outcomes for patients.

Can the Market Work?

The Congressional Budget Office (CBO) estimates that total prescription drug spending by and for the elderly will total at least $1.5 trillion in the decade from 2002 to 2011. In 1999, over 25 percent of Medicare beneficiaries had out-of-pocket drug expenses greater than $500.[16] In 2002, over 25 percent of beneficiaries had out-of-pocket drug expenses of more than $1,000.[17] Five percent were spending $4,000 or more out of pocket. These figures would be even higher if they took into account the related costs of premiums for insurance policies that cover drugs. Whether consumers are paying a larger or smaller share of total drug expenses, their actual cost burden has been increasing.

Considering the low incomes of many people on Medicare, it is no wonder that social service organizations tell stories of clients on Medicare who are forced to choose between filling prescriptions and buying groceries or paying their electricity bills.[18] Skipping doses and leaving prescriptions unfilled are common, but they tend to be more common among those without prescription drug insurance. In 2001, one study showed that 35 percent of the uninsured economized by skipping, compared to 22 percent of the insured.[19] Other studies show smaller percentages. Data from the Medicare Current Beneficiary Survey show that most people at least fill their prescriptions, but the survey does not address the prevalence of skipping doses.[20]

Few reliable studies have been done to determine how drug coverage influences actual health outcomes. A 1991 study of elderly Medicaid enrollees discovered a significantly greater increase in nursing-home admissions in states without drug coverage, along with some increase in hospitalizations.[21] In the same study, schizophrenic patients without drug coverage showed an increased use of emergency services and hospitalizations.

People on Medicare often pay twice as much for prescription drugs as drug manufacturers' most favored customers. Federal health authorities for the military and veterans negotiate the largest discounts for bulk purchases,[22] but under current law Medicare cannot negotiate the same deals. As private enterprises, pharmaceutical companies can legally sell the same drugs to different buyers at different prices. Variable pricing is protected by laws that make resale illegal, along with indirect discounting methods, like rebates, that are granted to health plans or state purchasers rather than pharmacies. Insurers may secure lower prices from pharmaceutical companies in exchange for putting their drugs on the insurers' formularies, from which contracted physicians are encouraged to prescribe. Foreign governments also negotiate lower prices for national distribution, a situation that has created growing interest in importing drugs from Canada. For manufacturers, bulk discounts represent an acceptable tradeoff between price and volume; for customers with less negotiating power, they lead to higher costs. Those who lose out are pri-

marily the uninsured and people on Medicare who do not have supplemental insurance. In the new Medicare Advantage arrangements, private
companies can negotiate prices even though traditional Medicare cannot.

In theory, MMA should provide the nearly forty million Medicare enrollees with enormous bargaining power. However, the law does not
allow Medicare to engage in centralized price negotiations, like those
used by the Veterans Administration, to lower the price of drugs. Further,
it prohibits the reimportation of drugs from countries paying lower costs,
such as Canada, unless the Secretary of the Department of Health and
Human Services guarantees the safety of the imported drugs.

The pharmaceutical industry's national association, Pharmaceutical
Research and Manufacturers of America (PhRMA), spends hundreds of
millions of dollars each year to promote their interests among policy makers. Medicare beneficiaries should have access to competitive prices without defeating the ability of the industry to make a profit. The questions
are how much profit is warranted and what type of consumer purchasing
power should be fostered.

The Drug Business

In an ideal market, prices eventually wind up modestly above the marginal cost of the product, meaning the cost of making one more unit is
somewhat less than the price it is sold for; the difference between marginal cost and price is the manufacturer's profit. Prescription drugs are
not priced anywhere near their marginal cost, because they are bought
and sold in unconventional ways. The principal factor complicating market forces for pharmaceutical drugs is the cost of research and development. On average it requires an estimated investment of $500 million and
more than eight years to bring a drug from inception to FDA approval
and use at the bedside. The cost includes investments in unsuccessful
drugs as well as the opportunity cost of money tied up in the development process. For this reason, new prescription drugs are protected by
patent. Until the patent expires, competitors and generic manufacturers
are prevented from duplicating the product.

The cost of manufacturing drugs once they are developed is typically
very low, and unregulated competition would drive the costs of new
drugs down dramatically. Patent protection is intended to protect the intellectual investment required to create and develop new drugs and sus-

tain the motivation for innovation. Granting exclusive property rights gives pharmaceutical companies a period of considerable market power over newly developed drugs. Changes in drug patent law in 1984 and further small adjustments in the 1990s have dramatically increased the term of exclusivity. One estimate shows the effective patent life of drugs increasing from about eight years in the early 1980s to more than fifteen years in the late 1990s.[23]

To extend their exclusive rights to highly profitable medications, pharmaceutical companies have become adept at manipulating the system: by incrementally changing an existing drug, revising the recommendations for its use, or altering the manufacturing process to renew its patent and maintain market share; by suing generic manufacturers to discourage entry into the market and suing states to discourage formulary systems that would force competition; or by narrowly defining the clinical scope of a drug to restrict its use to a prospective population under 200,000, which qualifies it for "orphan" drug status with extended patent privileges. Orphan drugs are used to treat rare conditions, so the market offers little financial incentive for companies to develop these drugs without special government protection. Actual uses for an orphan drug may be expanded later at the discretion of physicians.

Patent protection gives pharmaceutical companies the ability to set retail prices as they see fit, with high profits the inevitable result. Legitimate concerns about intellectual property rights make reform difficult, but critics are questioning the fairness of the current system. Among other proposals, some experts advocate shortening the length of pharmaceutical patents as a "free-market alternative to price controls."[24]

Market Failure and Its Remedies

Another reason that the free market fails to operate for prescription drugs is the lack of information and choice available to consumers. Apart from well-publicized excursions by busloads of elders shopping for drugs in Canada or Mexico, and growing Internet sales, most individuals do not have the resources or the opportunity to shop around for their prescription drugs. Manufacturer discounts typically apply not to the individual pharmacy but to insurance plans or health-care groups. In cases where an insurer pays, neither the physician nor the patient may know what the prescribed medications really cost. Third-party payment skews incentives for either patient or physician to economize.

Improving consumer choice, however, is not a solution because patients lack extensive medical knowledge. Moreover, personal circumstances make consumers' health-care purchasing decisions less elastic than choices about other market commodities. It is natural to defer to authority when dealing with something as vital as one's health; even physicians are hesitant about intervening in the clinical judgments involved in their own treatment when they happen to be patients.[25] Current trends are expecting patients to be discriminating consumers in all aspects of care, not only as purchasers of medication. Shopping around for medical treatment may be impossible when one's condition is urgent; or it may be unacceptable because of the patient's fear of losing or alienating the professional on whom he or she has come to rely.

The idea of market failure due to incomplete information, by itself, suggests a straightforward solution involving reforms that allow consumers access to the resources they need to make informed decisions. However, one reason why incomplete information has been tolerated for so long is a lack of interest or experience in acting like a consumer when one's health is at stake. Many patients want to be able simply to trust their doctor's advice.

Moreover, because of the vital importance of health, consumers are disinclined to argue about its price. As a society, too, we are uneasy about explicitly denying necessary care to anyone on the basis of inability to pay. This characteristic clearly distinguishes health care from normal market goods. Incomplete information about price can be tolerated because it is essentially irrelevant to the one clear goal of regaining one's health.

FORMULARIES

If the end consumer is not able or willing to make informed, price-sensitive decisions about prescription drugs, then how can the health-care system be organized to do so? Alain Enthoven suggests that purchasing decisions in health care require a third party to intervene between seller and buyer.[26] One example of a third-party arrangement is the drug formulary. For prescription drugs, physicians generate demand, but a separate group evaluates the equivalence and cost-effectiveness of the various alternatives available. It ranks comparable medications by their effectiveness and cost, sometimes limiting payment only to medications whose proven value justifies the cost. This is where the problem of third-party payment actually becomes part of the solution, by shifting the locus of responsibility.

Recognizing that both patient and physician have other concerns that make shopping around a low priority, the third party becomes the direct consumer responsible for upholding normal market relations, acquiring information and negotiating for the best deals. Health-care payers are already establishing drug formularies that rely on a group of medical experts to ascertain the most cost-effective treatments for various conditions. The selected drugs are then placed on a preferred list. When a new drug comes on the market, evidence is examined to see whether the drug is a significant improvement over existing medications. In some systems, physicians must obtain approval before prescribing a drug outside the formulary.

Many health plans and some state Medicaid programs are using or moving toward formularies. In the "preferred-drug" formulary recently established by the state of Oregon, information is posted on the cost-effectiveness of drugs in several classes.[27] Physicians are free to prescribe as they like, so long as they supply a reason for choosing higher-priced drugs when billing Medicaid. Several other states are following Oregon's example.[28] Other states require preauthorization for off-formulary prescriptions. Typically, when an off-formulary drug is prescribed, the patient pays any cost difference.

Large health-care systems in the United States, including State Medicaid programs, the Veterans Health Administration (VA) and a number of private systems, have implemented formularies in an attempt to achieve cost savings without jeopardizing health outcomes. A recent study by the Institute of Medicine (IOM) examined the VA formulary and the process for establishing it and concluded the system is a successful evidence-based practice that does not deny patients medically beneficial treatments.[29]

A formulary could enable Medicare to obtain the best prices for prescription drugs. The system should give pharmaceutical companies an incentive to offer reduced prices in order to place their drugs on the formulary list. With a Medicare formulary, the sales volume would be extraordinarily high, providing a strong incentive for companies to offer competitive prices.

Creating a fair, cost-effective, and medically sound formulary for Medicare would require analysis and discussion among experts in a variety of fields, including physicians, pharmacists, economists, business leaders, and beneficiaries. Technical questions of how to compare classes and doses of drugs, whether to use "reference pricing" (price compared to equally effective, often less costly or generic, drugs) as a standard, and other such complexities pale in comparison to the political firestorm bound to ignite with a proposal for a Medicare formulary.[30] Nonetheless, it is hard to argue against using systematic medical research to decide how best to spend taxpayer dollars on medical care. Overall, the approach appears sound in the way it adjusts the current system of market failure with a system that balances purchasing power, establishes the responsibility of knowledgeable providers, and maximizes information and discernment.

Among the issues to be addressed before adopting a formulary on such a large scale is the effect of such a plan on industry initiative. If patented drugs must compete in the market against less expensive generic drugs, or even against each other, will the value of patents decline to the point of hurting the pharmaceutical industry's incentive to conduct research? What level of competition is tolerable, considering the ongoing value of innovation?

PROTECTING INNOVATION

PhRMA argues that patent privileges and the high retail prices of prescription drugs are justified by the industry's costly investment in research and development (R&D), estimated at more than $20 billion per year.[31] The group warns that any action to curb the industry's profits would reduce incentives to conduct R&D, thereby damaging patients' interests. This argument is known as the "innovation threat." While it is true that R&D for effective new medications is a costly and time-consuming endeavor, how much money the industry actually invests or how badly it would be hurt if Medicare negotiated lower prices for medications are matters of debate.

One indicator involves a "reasonable pricing" policy established in 1989 by the National Institutes of Health (NIH) for cooperative R&D projects with private industry, rewarding the level of NIH (taxpayer) investment with a demand to set reasonable (affordable) prices for the resulting products. By 1995, NIH concluded that the policy was obstructing industry collaboration and abolished it. Within two years the number of new cooperative research agreements jumped from 32 to 153.[32] Congressional initiatives in 2001 and 2002 to reinstate a reasonable pricing policy stalled without results. Drug company influence in Congress prevailed.

The pharmaceutical industry regularly posts the highest profits of any sector in the health-care industry, and, in recent years, has showed the highest profitability of all industries. In 1999, it posted a 19 percent median return on revenues.[33] Nobody wants to curtail the industry's ability to finance R&D, but the question naturally arises whether such incentives are not already more than sufficient.

Not all R&D money is spent on researching breakthrough drugs for serious illnesses. Indeed, big drug companies are concerned that there are few real breakthroughs in their pipelines. Some R&D funds are spent on marketing research, and some on "me-too" or "copycat" drugs—drugs that are very similar to those of competitors. Me-too drugs allow a company to benefit financially from another company's research, as it is much cheaper to develop a drug when a similar drug already exists. Enthusiasm for copying drugs without adding value would probably subside under a formulary regime in which drugs are grouped by effectiveness and ranked by price.

In current pharmaceutical research, new drugs are designed on the basis of advances in biological research that suggest possibilities for medical intervention. From 1989 to 2000, the U.S. Food and Drug Administration approved an average of 86 drugs per year. About one-sixth, or thirteen drugs per year, contained new ingredients and demonstrated a clinical improvement over existing products; another 11 percent were identical to existing drugs. Half of the approved drugs involved only small modifications, like dosage or combination of ingredients, which allow a company to extend patent protection.

A large amount of cutting-edge research is funded by American taxpayers. NIH funds research in basic science at universities, medical schools, and other private and nonprofit institutions. Congress expanded the NIH budget tremendously in the past decade, from $10 billion in 1993 to more than $23 billion in 2002. Most of the money is disbursed in extramural grants for medical and biological research.[34] Academic and government researchers frequently license their preliminary findings to pharmaceutical companies, who then finance the further studies needed to gain FDA approval. In these cases, a breakthrough scientific discovery has already been made by the time a pharmaceutical company invests any money. Any argument that risk justifies the industry's level of profits is diminished by this publicly supported research platform, which provides a major springboard for innovation.

Often new drugs genuinely improve health outcomes, reducing mortality and morbidity, and reducing total health-care spending.[35] Innovation, however, can also be harmful, producing unexpected side effects or marginal benefits not justified by the extra expense. Encouraging the prosperity of the pharmaceutical industry with the right degree of moderation and responsibility is in everyone's interest.

Prescription Drug Benefits under MMA

MMA provides for the largest benefit expansion in Medicare's history: the new drug benefit is estimated to cost $410 billion between 2004 and 2013. The MMA has also changed the structure of the benefit in significant ways, most notably through the use of standalone plans to administer it and by prohibiting beneficiaries from buying supplemental plans to fill in significant gaps in coverage.

The new prescription drug benefit has been described as having a "doughnut hole" because there is a gap in coverage that must be filled by out-of-pocket spending before a patient becomes eligible for catastrophic coverage. Specifically, in addition to the monthly premium for Part D coverage, estimated to be $35 in 2006, the standard benefit will require the beneficiary to pay every year:

· the first $250 in drug costs (a deductible);

· 25 percent of total drug costs between $250 and $2,250;

· 100 percent of costs between $2,250 and $5,100; and

· the greater of $2 (for generics) or $5 (for brand-name drugs), or 5 percent coinsurance for each prescription.

The hole in the doughnut refers to the benefit gap of $2,850 for drug costs between $2,250 and $5,100. Before the beneficiary can qualify for catastrophic coverage, he or she will actually have to spend a total of $3,600: a $250 deductible, a copayment of 25 percent for amounts between $250 and $2,250, and the doughnut-hole amount of $2,850. This benefit gap will grow because deductibles, benefit limits, and catastrophic thresholds are indexed and will increase as Part D spending increases; beneficiaries are not likely to see a comparable increase in their incomes. For 2013, the benefit gap is estimated at $5,066.

This feature of MMA reduces protection against drug expenses just at the time when people with chronic conditions most need assistance to pay for medications. Many older people with chronic conditions take several medications and spend between $3,000 and $5,000 each year to maintain their quality of life and prevent loss of function.

Beneficiaries cannot avoid the doughnut hole and become eligible for the catastrophic coverage by purchasing a supplementary insurance policy. The new law requires out-of-pocket spending of $3,600 by the beneficiary, his or her family, or a state pharmaceutical program in order to qualify for catastrophic drug coverage. The rationale for this feature seems to be to control costs by making it difficult for beneficiaries to qualify. By requiring such large out-of-pocket expenditures, MMA may be discouraging inappropriate use of drugs—or creating the risk that people who truly need medications will do without. From the perspective of geriatric care, this is a short-sighted policy that will ultimately lead to higher costs and a lower quality of life for many Medicare recipients.

Beneficiaries who prefer to remain with the traditional, fee-for-service Medicare must enroll in a private prescription drug plan (PDP). If a PDP is not available in their area, Medicare will contract with a "fallback" plan to provide a benefit. Beneficiaries can also choose to enroll in an integrated Medicare Advantage program, which provides all Medicare benefits, including drugs. The precise costs and benefits of each plan may vary, although all plans are required to provide drugs in each therapeutic category, such as "lipid lowering," "antihypertensive," "diabetic," "antibiotic."

Many Medicare recipients will be faced with a bewildering array of choices among plans and types of coverage. Thus far only limited resources have been devoted to educating older people about the decisions they must make. Recent surveys indicate that most Medicare recipients do not understand the MMA and are confused about its provisions. Fewer than one in three seniors has ever accessed the Internet, which has been the primary source of information about the legislation. As the 2006 implementation date approaches, the need for clear and accessible information will increase.

ASSISTANCE FOR LOW-INCOME BENEFICIARIES

Beneficiaries with low incomes and limited assets will be eligible for additional assistance under the MMA. According to the Congressional Budget Office, as many as 14.7 million people may be eligible. Of this number, 6.4 million are "dual eligibles"—that is, eligible for both Medicaid and Medicare. Eligibility for the drug benefit is based on both income (it is restricted to people with an income less than 150 percent of the poverty level) and assets (currently pegged at $6,000 per individual and $9,000 per couple for beneficiaries with income below 135 percent of the poverty level, and $10,000 per individual or $20,000 per couple for incomes between 135 and 150 percent.) The complexity and difficulty of the qualification process and the reluctance of many older people to be labeled as poor will probably discourage some eligible people from taking advantage of this benefit.

Older people who are "dual eligibles" will begin to receive drug bene-fits under Medicare, rather than Medicaid, beginning in 2006. They will have to enroll in Part D plans to receive drug benefits. States, which bear about half the cost of Medicaid programs, will have to pay Medicare the amount they would have had to spend to provide drug benefits for this group—in a provision called the "clawback"—which will be about $88.5 billion between 2006 and 2013. If states want to provide additional assis-tance with cost sharing or an expanded formulary, they may do so only with state dollars, not with federal Medicaid matching funds.

National Politics

Congress has slowly expanded Medicare's drug coverage through the years by legislating coverage for specific drugs. Incremental change is po-litically easier to accomplish. Ironically, beneficiaries who cannot afford the prescription drugs necessary to manage a chronic condition at home and wind up in the hospital as a result find that Medicare will pay for in-patient drugs, in addition to other procedures that might have been pre-vented by good care management. The lack of comprehensive drug cov-erage clearly encourages more expensive treatments. Similarly, Medicare will pay for certain blood treatments, like erythropoietin given by injec-tion to keep up immune defenses and energy during chemotherapy, only if the patient goes into the hospital for the shots. The shots could easily be given at home, but they are not covered in that setting. Rules like this make no clinical or financial sense.

PhRMA and its body of industry giants are the top spenders in lobby-ing Congress, followed closely by the insurance industry.[36] In response to President Clinton's plan, announced in June 1999, to "modernize and strengthen Medicare for the twenty-first century," in part by adding a pre-scription drug benefit, the drug industry spent a record $262 million in the 1999–2000 election cycle to oppose the proposition with a combination of lobbying, campaign contributions, and issue ads. Incredibly, 625 lob-byists were hired, more than one for every member of Congress. One fea-ture of this blitz involved financing for a front organization called Citizens for Better Medicare, created and staffed by PhRMA, to run issue ads cost-ing about $65 million. An additional $10 million was funneled to the U.S. Chamber of Commerce to run ads attacking a Medicare drug benefit.

Curiously, some analysts and even certain leaders in the drug industry have suggested that a Medicare drug benefit could be a long-term advantage to pharmaceutical companies. Even if obliged to charge lower prices for drugs, the industry would make up the difference on expanded volume. This reasoning may explain why a few companies, such as the industry leader Merck, have been more supportive of a Medicare drug benefit. Merck already has an affiliate, Merck-Medco, that provides pharmaceutical benefits management to a large number of subscribers, mostly health insurers. The company profits from high-volume sales of both brand-name and generic drugs that correspond to formulary lists and is beginning to make use of systematic reviews of cost-effectiveness.

Medicare drug coverage will remain a topic of vigorous debate in Congress, as MMA 2003 is both costly and inadequate. It was a complicated mixture of agreements between different ideologies and different interest groups. Like the original Medicare legislation in 1965, it includes high payments to numerous interest groups (including physicians, hospitals, insurance companies, and drug companies); yet these enormous outlays will not provide the coverage to patients that people hoped for.

One of the strangest bills introduced in Congress in 2000 was the Prescription Drug Reimportation Act. The law would have allowed foreign companies that buy drugs from American pharmaceutical companies at discount prices to sell them back to U.S. consumers at prices below the typical U.S. retail cost. The act was not implemented because of concerns over ensuring the safety of the drugs, raised first by the Health and Human Services secretary Donna Shalala and later endorsed by her successor Tommy Thompson, with support from the FDA. This concern added credence to PhRMA's opposition to the bill all along. In any case, a market fix of this sort to reduce drug prices by a small degree would not supply the insurance coverage truly needed by Medicare beneficiaries. Nevertheless, support for this idea is strong among a bipartisan group of governors facing intense pressure from their citizens and from their state budgets to control the cost of prescription drugs.

The ideal way to incorporate a drug benefit in Medicare would be through a universal plan for all beneficiaries, regardless of income. The best solution would integrate the benefit into a newly rationalized system for the entire Medicare package, adhering to current knowledge in medical science and to the principles of geriatric medicine. The plain goal should be to maintain function and productivity among as many elders as possible. MMA adds a prescription-drug benefit without modernizing the rest of Medicare, which was the most politically feasible short-term solution. Following is a discussion of a number of underlying principles evident in this political debate, which is sure to continue.

PUBLIC VERSUS PRIVATE RESPONSIBILITY

Many policy makers favor establishing a drug benefit administered by the federal government under traditional Medicare. One of Medicare's advantages as an insurance program is its large pool of enrollees, which diversifies risk. Such a risk pool allows the healthy to support the costs of the unhealthy, so that the few people who incur astronomical health-care expenses are balanced by the majority of beneficiaries who have relatively modest needs. This is the ideal of any insurance system: everyone enjoys the assurance of coverage without feeling they are paying too much. Further, a program with a very large pool of beneficiaries should be able to leverage substantial price reductions with pharmaceutical companies. And because Medicare enjoys relatively low administrative costs, adding a new benefit to the existing program should not be as costly as creating new programs from scratch.

Despite these advantages, the ideological fear of the government "setting prices" led policy makers to favor options to privatize the drug benefit. Private insurers compete to attract enrollees just as Medicare+Choice plans previously did, arguing that consumers benefit from additional choice in plan designs—although in fact traditional Medicare allows the widest choice among doctors and hospitals. The argument for "choice" can be misleading. Critics point out that private plans add another layer of bureaucracy and therefore of cost. Initially, there was not much interest among private insurers in accepting the risk of offering drug coverage to elders, because they see the large costs in their commercial plans and fear the risk of adverse selection; but they were offered financial incentives to do so, adding to the cost of the MMA without adding to the benefits for seniors.

Time will tell whether these market solutions will create effective coverage for seniors. The private plans have to worry about their bottom lines, and the for-profit companies have to satisfy shareholders. Providing good medication coverage will tend to attract patients with chronic illness, who need more drugs and other expensive services. Because this adverse selection did not work for previous Medicare programs, it is hard to see why Medicare Advantage should fare any better. Requirements for private plans to accept large regional populations, rather than select for healthier patients, are already being resisted by the health-care industry.

The fundamental problem with breaking up Medicare is that market segmentation leads to the practice of risk selection by commercial plans. When Germany planned its new provision of insurance for long-term care in 1994, for example, rather than assume that the private market promised the best solution, legislators consulted private insurers. When the private market rejected the opportunity, Germany created a government insurance program.[37] Long-term care is as troublesome for private administration as prescription drugs are. Leaders who advocate reliance on market forces prefer the idea of raising financial incentives for private insurers until they finally say yes and agree to enter the Medicare market. One wonders how such intervention can produce an efficient and sustainable program. Although drug companies flourish under this model, everyone else suffers: not only individual patients, but insurance companies, hospitals, health plans, and state governments.

UNIVERSAL BENEFIT VERSUS NEED-BASED ELIGIBILITY

Because we will all benefit from Medicare at some point, and most of us have family members who currently rely on it, the program enjoys a high profile with extraordinary popular support. Needs-based programs reserved for the poor, like Medicaid, tend to carry a social stigma and are too often underfunded. Large sectors of the population receive no direct benefit and therefore find few reasons to invest in the success of such programs.

Apart from weaker social and political support, many other problems beset programs that define eligibility through means tests or asset tests. For one thing, a means test for health benefits is considered unacceptably demeaning in many other countries. The administrative and personal burden of proving poverty adds to cost and hassle for patients. Some programs ease the burden by allowing self-declaration rather than documented proof.[38] Second, means testing creates perverse incentives to stay poor or become poor in order to qualify. Economists identify this kind of change in behavior, due to distinctions in the tax system, as inefficient, producing a "deadweight loss." For some reason they are less vocal with regard to means tests. Yet examples of inefficiency abound. To qualify for Medicaid coverage of long-term care, patients must first "spend down" their assets, effectively becoming impoverished in order to become eligible. In Australia, a means-tested pension program resulted in workers' spending down before retirement in order to qualify, a trend that finally led the government to institute a universal system.[39] Third, the application of a means test creates uncertainty about eligibility that results in many eligible people not participating. Fourth, and of most concern in health care, a means test imposes discontinuity in care if income fluctuates or eligibility rules are changed, as individuals move in and out of eligibility. Currently, primary care and mental-health services, as well as care management of chronic illness, are disrupted as coverage changes.[40]

Since before Medicare was enacted, tension has existed between those who support a social-insurance health program for older citizens and those who prefer to limit the federal government's role in social programs, including health insurance. While some argue that the best way to spread the financial risk of a drug benefit is to enroll all Medicare beneficiaries regardless of income, others argue that any new benefit should be limited to those who cannot otherwise afford it. Some are advancing the same means-test idea for Social Security. In spite of the obvious burdens and disadvantages of a means test, the debate is by no means resolved and will certainly be heard repeatedly in the coming years.

DEFINED BENEFIT VERSUS DEFINED CONTRIBUTION

The 1998–1999 Bipartisan Commission on the Future of Medicare, which was appointed by President Clinton to create a Medicare program that would work for the future, disbanded unsuccessfully in part because of the intense philosophical disagreement between members who wanted to retain Medicare's defined-benefit structure and those who wanted to transform Medicare into a defined-contribution plan. Currently, everyone on Medicare is entitled to the same clearly defined benefits. Even Medicare HMOs are required to provide a certain set of basic Medicare benefits, although they can add additional benefits and decide when and how enrollees receive them. Some in Congress favor a shift to a defined-contribution plan, in which the government would allot each person on Medicare a defined sum (like a voucher) with which to shop among different Medicare plans—presumably mostly private plans, with a government-run option.

Prescription drugs are an important part of this discussion. In a contribution system, those who needed many prescription drugs could choose a plan that offers drug coverage, while those with fewer health needs could choose a less expensive plan that offered more limited benefits. Such a scheme enhances flexibility in a normal market, but insurance is not a normal market. Segmenting the population into low and high risks would make policies unaffordable for those who need them most. The proposal to expand choice for drug coverage could destroy the social-insurance concept that has made Medicare so strong and so popular for more than thirty-five years.

In the insurance industry, *adverse selection* refers to a situation where only those with high risks purchase policies, and those with low risks drop out. In today's private market for health insurance, carriers must always worry about competitors offering lower-priced policies to draw away the low risks. When this happens, a carrier may be forced to raise premiums to cover the increased costs of the high risks, whereupon more low-risk clients drop out, premiums rise again, and so on, creating a death spiral for the carrier. This phenomenon is exactly the issue facing Medicare managed care: it is the reason that many Medicare+Choice plans withdrew from the market. With drug benefits in particular, adverse selection is a serious concern.

In a universal-benefit program like Medicare, the problem of adverse selection does not exist. The gravest danger in shifting Medicare towards a defined-contribution model is that it would open the door to adverse risk selection. Medicare would take on the attributes of the fragmented system of private health insurance, in which insuring the people who need coverage most becomes prohibitively expensive.

Moreover, people are not very prescient about future risks. If a relatively healthy seventy-year-old man chooses to avoid the high premiums of a comprehensive plan and opts for a limited low-cost plan, and then develops serious heart disease or cancer, he cannot then switch to a higher-benefit plan: the carrier will deny him coverage because of his preexisting condition. He will spend all of his personal assets on health care, turn to his family for assistance, and then become impoverished and dependent on Medicaid. This is exactly the situation that led to the creation of traditional Medicare in 1965. Widely shared risk with defined benefits remains more efficient, fair, and sustainable.

INTEREST-GROUP POLITICS

Despite the medical arguments for affordable prescription drugs, the issue might not have reached the political limelight without the efforts of advocacy organizations for older people. Many interest groups for the aging have put health care at the top of their agendas and vigorously supported a prescription-drug benefit. Some staged media events showing their members taking buses to Canada or Mexico to buy American-made drugs at lower prices. Other groups have issued policy reports documenting their members' and clients' needs for prescription drugs.

In March 2000, OWL (the Older Women's League) released a report titled *Prescription for Change: Why Women Need a Medicare Drug Benefit*.

In July 2000, Families USA released *Cost Overdose: Growth in Drug Spending for the Elderly, 1992–2010,* in addition to its annual *Still Rising* reports on the increasing costs of prescription drugs. These reports bring consumers' needs and experiences to the attention of policy makers and the media. These efforts will not be stilled by the passage of the 2003 MMA because the problem is not yet solved.

Consumer groups are not, of course, the only interest groups in Washington involved in the prescription-drug debate. Citizens for a Better Medicare, a front organization for PhRMA, posed as a consumer group to lobby against a drug benefit through extensive television advertising. One of the group's television commercials featured a woman named Flo asking the government to please "stay out of my medicine cabinet." The misleading message was that with a Medicare drug benefit, the government would control access to medications. Although some limits would have to be applied to a Medicare drug benefit, probably through an evidence-based formulary, the list of choices would certainly be extensive; and the few drugs not covered would still be available, probably by the patients' paying the difference between the cost for the drug and that for a similar formulary drug or through supplementary insurance policies. Sharply focused on defeating a Medicare drug benefit, the ads were well-funded, pervasive, and effective in frightening people. Once the legislation included prohibitions against evidence-based programs and Medicare negotiated prices, the drug industry supported the bill.

Some health-care providers supported PhRMA's position. Although some provider groups, especially primary-care physicians, recognized the importance of affordable medications and expressed support for a Medicare drug benefit, other groups lobbied against it for fear it would disrupt scheduled increases in their Medicare-approved fees.[41] With health-care providers, interest groups, and politicians lining up on different sides of the prescription-drug debate, the outcome will be more complicated than a simple yes-or-no proposition. In any case, MMA represents not the end of the debate but the beginning of a new process to define the Medicare system.

CONGRESS AND INCREMENTAL COVERAGE CHANGES

Congress occasionally gets a notion that Medicare should cover some specific condition or treatment and passes a law for it, even if it forces an exception to established Medicare law. In 1972, for example, Congress passed a law enabling people with end-stage renal disease (ESRD) to receive full Medicare coverage, including full coverage of dialysis, regardless of age. The dramatic, lifesaving technology was demonstrated with a live patient in the House of Representatives. Subsequent benefit additions have not been as sweeping as the ESRD benefit, partly because the experience there has proved so much more costly than originally projected.

Under traditional Medicare legislation, drugs are covered when received as part of inpatient treatment, either in a hospital or nursing home; when they must be administered by a physician (these are covered under Medicare Part B when administered by a physician or member of his/her office staff); or when they are administered through pumps recognized as durable medical equipment (DME). In the last instance, coverage (under Part B) applies to both ambulatory infusion pumps and stationary equipment used in the patient's home but does not extend to disposable pumps, which are not considered DME.

In 1983, Congress added a Medicare hospice benefit (see chapter 5) that includes coverage for outpatient prescription drugs for patients who qualify. Normally, outpatient drugs have not been covered, but exceptions were made as part of the hospice benefit and for drugs in the categories listed below. These are examples of how Congressional micromanagement responds to special needs but doesn't create a workable insurance plan for most people. Over recent years Medicare began to cover the following outpatient prescription drugs:

Injectable drugs administered by a physician.   Since the late 1960s, Medicare has covered drugs that need to be administered in a physician's office. In the Omnibus Budget Reconciliation Act (OBRA) of 1990, Medicare drug coverage was expanded to include injectable drugs for the treatment of osteoporosis for patients who are unable to administer the drugs themselves or who meet the requirements for Medicare home health care.

Why was this medication covered while other injectable drugs were not? Congress likely wanted to be seen to make Medicare more responsive to women's needs, and public awareness of the dangers of osteoporosis had increased. The exception illustrates the fragmented approach that too often determines Medicare coverage rules.

Later, in the Consolidated Appropriations Act of 2000, Congress prohibited Medicare from making "any regulation or other transmittal or policy directive that has the effect of imposing a restriction on the coverage of injectable drugs."[42] Consequently, coverage of this category of drugs was expanded. CMS has instructed contractors how to distinguish drugs that can be self-administered; these are not covered. Considering the pressure senior groups have put on Congress to expand Medicare drug coverage, it is probably no coincidence that Congress was lenient in expanding coverage to the classification of injectable drugs during an election year.

Drugs used in chemotherapy.   Any health-care insurance that controls costs by imposing conditions and exclusions risks creating a trend for expensive services that are covered to be overused at the expense of less costly alternatives that are not covered. This situation arose with chemotherapy drugs. Since Medicare did not generally pay for home or self-administered drugs but did pay for drugs received in the hospital, cancer patients were going to the hospital to obtain intravenous forms of their chemotherapy treatments, even when oral forms were available.

In 1991, the General Accounting Office documented that "Medicare reimbursement policies prevented cancer patients from receiving the full benefits of cancer research."[43] The report motivated Representative Sander Levin (D-Mich.), on the House Ways and Means Committee, to introduce a bill called the Medicare Cancer Coverage Improvement Act of 1991. The Act provided Medicare coverage for oral anticancer agents that can be substituted for injectable forms of the same drugs. Vetoed by the first President Bush, the bill was reintroduced in 1993 as part of the House budget bill and passed.

The Balanced Budget Act of 1997 expanded Medicare coverage, under certain conditions, to include an oral antiemetic drug used as part of an anticancer chemotherapy regime. The rationale was that an oral chemotherapy drug would not be effective without the complementary antiemetic drug. Current law provides for Medicare payment of both an oral chemotherapy drug and an oral antiemetic drug. These are exceptions to the general rule that Medicare does not pay for self-administered drugs. Unfortunately, the new benefits only apply to certain cancer patients. People with heart failure are another group especially dependent on self-administered drugs whose needs have not yet been recognized in this process of incremental reforms.

Exclusions to benefits can create perverse incentives. Medicare payment for chemotherapy drugs administered in physicians' offices, for example, created a financial boon for oncologists, who bill Medicare for administering chemotherapy drugs and also for the medications themselves, which may be supplied by the manufacturer at prices greatly reduced from the billing price. Case studies show that 50 percent to 66 percent of practice revenues for most oncologists derive from chemotherapy drugs and consequent patient evaluation and management.[44] Here again, special rules produce paradoxical incentives. The oncologist has much more incentive to give chemotherapy than to discuss other options with patients. Of course, aggressive cancer treatment may be appropriate, but the oncologist has a financial reason to avoid offering other options, like palliative care, that are generally not covered. Cancer patients may spend the last few weeks of their lives suffering the adverse effects of chemotherapy drugs rather than saying goodbye to loved ones and dying in comfort and dignity. New and expensive arthritis medications that are covered if administered in a doctor's office are creating the same incentives, leading to increased use of this alternative and the inability to access these drugs through home care programs.

Drugs associated with kidney dialysis.   In 1983, the drug Epogen (erythropoietin) was developed to help treat the anemia common in patients with chronic renal failure. In the 1980s, dialysis centers began administering erythropoietin (it must be injected) to patients and billing Medicare for the administration of the drug. Because there was no national law authorizing Medicare coverage for this drug, regional intermediaries exercised their discretion in determining what was medically necessary and began to pay for it. Claims for erythropoietin reimbursement grew throughout the 1980s. With OBRA 1990, Congress established a national payment and coverage policy for erythropoietin. As another exception to the rule that Medicare does not pay for self-administered drugs, Medicare now pays for erythropoietin administered in a dialysis facility or self-administered at home in cases of renal failure but does not pay for the drug in cases of chemotherapy-related anemia or other conditions for which the FDA has approved its use. To qualify for coverage, patients who need erythropoietin to counteract chemotherapy side effects must visit a doctor's office or go into the hospital. The result is a fee for a service the patient could just as well receive for free at home.

Drugs associated with organ transplants.   In 1984, the FDA approved the drug cyclosporine for immunosuppressive therapy in relation to organ transplants. In 1986, Congress approved Medicare coverage for immunosuppressants for one year after an organ transplant.[45] In 1988, the Medicare Catastrophic Coverage Act extended coverage beyond one year after a transplant, but the law was repealed a year later. In 1993, coverage of immunosuppressive drugs was extended again, eventually providing coverage for three years after a transplant. In 1999, coverage was extended another eight months. In 2000, restrictions were abolished altogether.[46] As of 2001, immunosuppressive drugs are covered for the lifetime of the organ.

The congressional debates on these changes focused on cost savings. Representative Doug Walgreen (D-Penn.) sponsored the original legislation for Medicare coverage of immunosuppressants largely on the basis of cost efficiency. The initial coverage of one year was clearly inadequate. Even in 1992, Medicare was paying $3.5 million per year to retransplant organs or to return patients to kidney dialysis in part because of limited immunosuppressive drug coverage.[47] The cost of providing appropriate drugs would have been only $464,000. In 1993, Congress heeded the data and voted for more cost savings. In doing so, it also increased the viability of organ transplants. As of 2002, dialysis cost $50,000 per year, whereas drug therapy cost approximately $8,000 per year.[48] The medical alternatives here provide a stark example of the health and economic benefits to be derived from extending Medicare drug coverage.

Vaccines.   Although Medicare generally does not pay for vaccines, three separate laws have been passed to make exceptions: pneumococcal vaccine in 1980, hepatitis B for high-risk individuals in 1984, and influenza in 1991. In these cases, Medicare pays for the vaccines and their administration.

An Appeal to Logic

Few would argue against any of these incremental coverage decisions for Medicare. A relevant question, however, is why Congress is the body making decisions about medical necessity. Oral cancer therapy, for example, is no more essential to life than oral diabetes, heart, or blood-pressure medicines, yet Medicare has not covered these other conditions. Episodic attention spurred by vocal interest groups and election politics results in laws that make inequitable and illogical distinctions.

Medicare is highly complicated and has many areas in which change could reduce costs and improve health, yet Congress has come nowhere near agreeing on major systemic reforms. Incremental reforms appear to be the best it can do. Sometimes the changes increase benefits, as with the extensions of drug benefits discussed above. At other times, the changes cut payments to providers, reducing available benefits. This kind of incrementalism will not give people on Medicare and their physicians the kind of flexibility they need for optimal treatment, but at least it shows that Congress sometimes listens and responds to the needs and concerns of the voting public. This should give the baby boomers encouragement as they move toward Medicare eligibility.

Ideally, decisions about medical necessity would not involve Congress at all. Congress needs to establish the general contours of appropriate health security and budget accountability, but authority for particular decisions of medical necessity needs to be entrusted to local medical providers. To make this arrangement work, however, CMS would first need to learn how to operate as a prudent purchaser of quality care, and Congress would need to commit to covering such care, protecting it as much as possible from the profit interests of the commercial health-care industry, as most other developed countries have managed to do.

If Congress really wants to establish a comprehensive drug benefit for Medicare, it could control costs by establishing a formulary that covers the most cost-effective drugs for each disease. This step could help Medicare control drug spending and avoid discriminating against people unfortunate enough to develop a disease for which Medicare does not currently cover the necessary drugs. It makes no logical or medical sense to cover drugs for some diseases and not for others. Politicians should not be making these decisions. Ideally, Medicare's entire benefits package should be restructured according to the principles of modern geriatric medicine, including care management and the monitoring of chronic conditions. Cost-effective, evidence-based use of prescription drugs is an essential aspect of this goal.

CHAPTER 10

Politics

Reforming Medicare Reform

Medicare has always been a highly political program. The substantial costs of providing health-care insurance for approximately forty million people with the greatest health needs draws close scrutiny from policy makers. Various interest groups advocate for their often competing agendas. Congress has the ability to change the fundamental features of Medicare as it chooses. The president can influence Medicare policy with administrative initiatives (but cannot implement major changes without support from Congress).

Ironically, some of those most closely involved with Medicare have the least input into how it works. Providers and beneficiaries are affected only when the definitions of benefits and procedures filter down to the intermediary organizations that contract to process claims for Medicare. The contractors are the front line of Medicare politics, but they "operate under very tight budget constraints, giving them few incentives to help providers and enrollees seeking clarification."[1] And because administrative expenses for Medicare are very low—less than 2 percent of all benefit payments—there is virtually no allowance for management and purchasing decisions or for coordination of care and education of providers and beneficiaries.

This lack of education has potentially disastrous consequences for patients. For example, more than one-third of the elderly surveyed in 1998 did not know that traditional Medicare did not cover prescription drugs.[2] More than half do not know that long-term nursing home care is not covered. Few understand the choices involved in Medicare managed care.

Policy changes are often difficult even for providers to comprehend, let alone the millions of older adults whose health care is affected. Many are not highly educated, and 10 to 20 percent have some type of cognitive impairment, such as Alzheimer's disease.[3] The 2003 Medicare legislation presents special challenges: a large majority of the elderly report confusion about elements of the law, particularly the coverage of prescription drugs.

Numerous piecemeal policies, shaped in the 1990s by the Balanced Budget Act of 1997, continue to remake Medicare. BBA radically changed the way Medicare reimburses many providers, expanded Medicare managed care, cut Medicare support for graduate medical education, and added several preventive benefits to the basic benefits package, including mammograms, colorectal and prostate screenings, and bone density scans. In 2003, the Medicare Prescription Drug Improvement and Modernization Act made major changes to the program, including not only the long-awaited prescription-drug benefit but also incentives for privatization intended to shift enrollees into HMOs and PPOs, the establishment of tax-sheltered Health Savings Accounts, the addition of new preventive benefits, and a range of cost-containment efforts.

In spite of some legislative tinkering with Medicare's features and structure, the period between its inception and 1994 was characterized by the politics of consensus.[4] Medicare was such a popular program that politicians were reluctant to suggest any fundamental changes. Democrats and Republicans agreed on the program's general direction, and Medicare policy making focused on small reforms rather than large-scale overhaul. Most important, there was a consensus on the program's value. In 1995, this consensus appeared to fracture, and Medicare entered a new era of fierce partisanship and disagreement. Today ideological politics is putting Medicare's basic structure and social-insurance philosophy up for debate. The 2003 legislation, which was the subject of fierce political and public controversy, has moved the program significantly in the direction of privatization.

As Congress continues to alter the Medicare program and new laws proliferate, one has to ask whether we are really making progress or simply stirring the pot to satisfy political interests. Could we avoid incremental reforms and decide instead on a wholesale reform that works better for all? Could Congress accomplish such a thing? Should Congress, in any case, be spending time on micromanaging these critical health-care decisions for us? And if Congress is not the appropriate body to manage

Medicare, what is? The political foundation of Medicare may need reform as much as other areas discussed earlier.

Medicare—The History of Political Forces

Huge government programs affecting millions of people will always stimulate political debate. The original Medicare legislation was also born of expediency and political compromise. In the early 1950s, when President Truman realized Congress would not pass his broad proposal for universal health care, he decided to focus his attention on health insurance for people receiving Social Security benefits. In 1950, Oscar Ewing, head of the Federal Security Agency, convened the National Conference on Aging. In the summer following the conference, Ewing announced Truman's proposal to deliver insurance coverage for sixty days of hospital care to the seven million aged Social Security recipients.

Social Security was a popular national institution that had overcome the public suspicion of government-funded social programs. In the 1930s, after the AMA opposed private health insurance (in the form of the early Blue Shield and Blue Cross plans) as a type of socialism, the expectation prevailed that physicians would charge what the market could bear, and people would pay out of pocket for services without interference by government or corporate intermediaries. AMA opposition prevented the inclusion of health insurance in the 1935 enactment of Social Security legislation. Later, many physicians came to agree that insurance was the only way to assure payment for increasingly expensive services, but the AMA continued to oppose any government involvement.

Truman's Medicare proposal was obstructed by fierce opposition from organized medicine, which linked the proposed health plan with Social Security and succeeded in making the idea look like social insurance rather than charity or welfare. Older Americans, however, were perceived as both needy and deserving, having, through no fault of their own, lower earnings and higher health costs than the general public. They were also much less likely to have employment-based or private insurance. Private insurers often excluded them as too expensive to insure or charged unaffordable premiums.

Delayed during the Eisenhower years, serious debate over Medicare did not begin in Congress until 1958, six years after Truman's proposal. In 1958 the precursor to today's Medicare Part A hospital insurance, the Forand Bill, was debated in the House Ways and Means Committee. The

AMA increased its lobbying budget fivefold that year to oppose the bill. Federal hospital insurance is "dangerous to the basic principles underlying our American system of medical care," the AMA argued, praising the free market as the basic principle of the U.S. system of medical care.[5] Many agreed. The Forand Bill was defeated in 1959.

The debate surrounding the bill hinged on three questions: Do all older citizens really need help paying for health insurance? Does a limited hospital benefit provide enough help to the needy? And how should the program be financed—by the federal or state governments? From today's perspective, these questions remain worth asking.

Between 1958 and 1965, the Senate Finance Committee held annual Medicare meetings at which hundreds of interest groups aired their views. Conservative leaders felt compelled to produce an alternative to the Forand Bill. They came up with a "welfare approach" in the Kerr-Mills Bill, introduced in 1960. Kerr-Mills was a means-tested program for people aged sixty-five and over with low incomes. It offered a comprehensive benefits package, complete with physician services, hospital and nursing-home care, and prescription drugs, paid for with matching state and federal funds, very much resembling today's Medicaid program. Kerr-Mills was enacted in 1960. Within three years, thirty-two states had begun programs, but only four were providing the full range of benefits described in the law. Most state programs imposed strict limits on eligibility and coverage.[6] From the beginning, the bill was recognized by lawmakers as inadequate for addressing the needs of elders.[7]

Although the AMA originally opposed the Kerr-Mills legislation, it reversed its position and endorsed the idea in 1961. Entering office that year, President Kennedy had pledged to enact a compulsory health-insurance law for all aged Social Security beneficiaries. To combat this measure, the AMA chose to back the Byrnes Bill, which offered insurance with subsidized monthly premiums to some older citizens. The plan expanded the range of benefits offered under Kerr-Mills but remained focused on poorer people and voluntary participation.

The AMA invested significant effort in trying to demonstrate that the majority of the elderly were well-off and did not need Medicare, claiming they already enjoyed employment-based benefits as well as opportunities for private insurance. A voluntary system, with a little help for the poor, was all that was necessary. This line of reasoning was contradicted by the insurance industry itself, which testified that insuring the elderly was generally a losing business. Equally spurious was the AMA prediction in 1961 that the costs of medical care would decline, obviating the need for public insurance because "scientific advances in medicine will enable us to safeguard the health of the elderly with increasing efficiency."[8] Although scientific medical advances have certainly improved the health and longevity of many citizens, costs are not declining but continue to rise steeply.

President Kennedy wrote that he favored a program grounded in the "sound and proven Social Security principles" because they were "one of the most popular approaches in America."[9] He appointed Wilbur J. Cohen, assistant secretary of the Department of Health, Education, and Welfare and an experienced Social Security reformer, to supervise the drafting of legislation, move it through Congress, and help with its implementation. In this capacity, Cohen devoted significant time and energy to courting members of Congress, including Wilbur Mills, chair of the House Ways and Means Committee, and other influential committee members.[10]

With Lyndon Johnson's landslide Democratic victory in 1964, it looked likely that a bill would be passed in 1965. Mills crafted a compromise that accommodated all the positions on the table and devised the three-tiered system we know today; for the elderly, Medicare Part A for hospital insurance, and Part B as a voluntary supplement for physician services; and, for all with low incomes, Medicaid, funded and administered in partnership with the states. In the end, seniors of all income levels and the poor of all ages were eligible for some type of government-sponsored health insurance.

SUCCESSFUL RESULTS

One of the great ironies often pointed out by policy analysts is that contrary to AMA expectations, physician incomes have dramatically increased since Medicare's enactment, in part because the expansion of insurance coverage has led to increased patient volume. This experience should reassure the pharmaceutical industry, which has opposed proposals to rationalize and expand drug coverage. Forty years ago organized medicine was trying to prevent Medicare; now it is focused on maintaining it.

Of course, part of the reason Medicare has benefited medical providers is that the final compromise incorporated many of the conditions stipulated by organized medicine, including physician exemption from fee schedules, with payment according to "reasonable and customary charges." As observed in chapter 8, the inflationary nature of this deal became obvious and ultimately untenable. Now the battles over resource-based relative-value fee schedules inspire extraordinary activity by specialty groups whose incomes are threatened. The system has significantly changed the ethos of the medical profession and created a large upper class of technology-based physicians whose primary source of income is Medicare. Increased wealth allows greater projections of political influence from many directions.

Paul Starr, in his classic work on the social history of the American medical profession, describes the enactment of Medicare as a "politics of accommodation." [11] Congress and the administration were eager to gain the support of physicians and hospitals. The best reason for creating a separate Part B insurance for physician services was to limit the effect of the great passions aroused in the medical profession over the administration of the program. Similarly, hospitals were offered generous payments based on "cost-plus" reimbursement, with adjustments that favored capital investment. As with physicians' fees, these payments inflated dramatically, leading to a boom in hospital construction, technology acquisition, capitalization, and for-profit enterprise.

With all its developments over forty years, Medicare remains an anomaly in the United States: a government-run, guaranteed health-insurance program for a segment of the population, all eligible for equal coverage because they have contributed to the economy throughout their working lives. Even Social Security, Medicare's nearest social-insurance relative, directs extra support to those at lower incomes. For income security, such an orientation is appropriate.

The uniformity of benefits for all under Medicare is an important reason for the program's strong public support. From the beginning, some policy makers have advocated means testing in Medicare; many others have argued against it because "giving benefits only to *some* of [the elderly] who meet an income test would change the character of the program from social insurance to 'welfare,' and would be perceived by Americans as 'humiliating' and 'undignified.' "[12]

By linking Medicare to Social Security, Medicare advocates were able to gain public support for Medicare despite widespread ambivalence or hostility toward the social-contract philosophy and government-administered programs. The idea of benefits for all inspires support. As regards health security, Medicare established a new value for uniformity, cementing a social contract between generations based on need. Distinguishing Medicaid as a separate program to support low-income health care avoided the need to include an income test and subsidies of some sort in Medicare.

Medicare was a political compromise, and the long-term implications of what care is covered and how claims are paid were not given the serious consideration they deserved. In any case, how to determine the effectiveness of medical care was not well understood at that time. Neither were the specialized knowledge of geriatric medicine, including the different demands of chronic care, or the ways in which structures of delivery systems and payment would influence overall costs. We have made considerable progress in these areas over the last thirty years and have much better ideas about how to manage a system to achieve the best results.

Politics in Motion

How does Congress get involved in micromanaging Medicare? Recent debates surrounding mammography reimbursement rates illustrate this phenomenon as well as the high levels of commitment by stakeholders to defend their financial turf. With BBA 1997, Congress expanded the preventive benefits covered by Medicare, including mammograms for preventive purposes, but maintained an earlier distinction in payment rates based on the reason for the mammogram. The "diagnostic mammogram," ordered only when a problem is suspected, was covered at a higher fee. The "screening mammogram" was compensated at a lower fee to discourage overuse.

Because BBA 1997 covered one annual mammogram for all women over age forty, overuse was no longer an issue, and the difference in reimbursement made no sense. Many radiologists who perform mammograms had long opposed the distinction for what amounted to the same procedure. The argument only gained strength once BBA increased the incentives for women to get regular mammograms. As the number of tests requested increased enormously, radiologists warned that low reimbursement rates were causing mammography centers to scale back services or close, making it impossible for many women to schedule timely mammogram appointments.[13]

As is usually the case in the politics of Medicare, whenever one group wants additional money, it is challenged by others who want their share of the pie. In this case, the American Association of Health Plans (AAHP) disputed the radiologists' claim that reimbursement rates were inadequate. Because private insurance companies frequently base their reimbursement rates on the amounts paid by Medicare, they have an interest in keeping their own mammogram reimbursement rates as low as possible.

At the 1998 meeting of the Radiology Society of North America, a panel of physicians warned that because of inadequate reimbursement rates from Medicare and other insurers and fears of malpractice claims (due to irreducible errors—the examinations miss 10 to 20 percent of cancers), some mammography centers were closing. With this argument, the Radiology Society sent a letter to HCFA trying to influence Congress to pay for mammograms according to the standard physician fee schedule. The letter warned that many physicians were choosing not to enter mammography fellowships, creating a shortage of qualified physicians.

The efforts paid off. The Modernization of Screening Mammography benefit was part of a large piece of legislation passed in the final months of the Clinton administration. Since 2002, screening mammograms have been paid for on the same basis as diagnostic mammograms. By vocally educating members of Congress about their concerns, radiologists and other groups helped rationalize Medicare's paradoxical laws and rules.

This story shows that public access to government can work to effect change. It is also a perfect example of "body-part health policy," with one concern addressed at a time, often in response to the demands of special-interest groups. Although the individual consequences of this process may appear constructive, as here, the overall result is a system of reimbursement more complex than the federal tax code. Multiply the individual interests involved by the time and money spent in lobbying, debating, and deciding, and one begins to wonder if there is not a way to determine Medicare reimbursement without involving the nation's top leaders in decisions that essentially result in the corporate practice of medicine—which Medicare was originally designed to avoid.

Senior Interests at Work

The compromise that created Medicare and Medicaid under the Social Security Act in 1965 merged all the alternatives in contention: social insurance with both mandatory and voluntary components, plus a separate means-tested program for the poor. Interestingly, the elderly and the poor were not the primary lobbying force behind this remarkable development.

Although Medicare is ostensibly a program dedicated to health security for older adults, it is also a huge payment program for health-care providers. We have already seen the central importance of physicians, represented by the AMA, in debates over legislation. Although membership began to decline in the mid-1950s, the AMA was still much stronger in 1965 than it is today and represented a larger proportion of American physicians than it does now. At the time, the AMA had the confidence and support of most American medical professionals and the commensurate lobbying influence.

In addition, the evident needs of older adults were a potent force on their own. From the New Deal until the end of the 1970s, older citizens were "compassionately stereotyped by the media as poor, frail, dependent, and above all, deserving."[14] This generally accepted image, and the voting public's overwhelming support of programs for seniors, encouraged Congress to enact Social Security, Medicare, the Older Americans Act, the Employee Retirement Income Security Act (ERISA), special tax exemptions and credits, and many other programs protecting citizens almost exclusively on the basis of age. Differences in income, race, health status, and social conditions were rarely addressed in these policies.

When Social Security and Medicare were established, aging interest groups were not yet an organized political force. Both programs were established through initiatives of political leaders and other professionals, not as a result of grassroots organizing. The voices heard by public officials were those of the adult children paying their parents' medical bills. Today, the voices of older citizens are heard loud and clear in Washington.

The Origins of AARP

The National Council of Senior Citizens for Health Care (NCSC) was the only major political group of older adults in the 1960s, and it was closely affiliated with the AFL-CIO rather than existing as an independent interest group.[15] AARP had not yet become a vocal entity, despite its membership of nearly one million in 1964.[16] The organization's origins were based in commercial interests selling health insurance, not political activism.

Ethel Percy Andrus, a retired teacher and activist, established the National Retired Teachers Association (NRTA) in 1947. NRTA focused on promoting continuous educational opportunity, promoting financial security in retirement, protecting the rights of citizens—especially of the elderly and children—promoting stable and healthy communities, and improving mental and physical health.[17]

By 1955, Andrus had started a convalescent village and retirement home for NRTA teachers but was unable to arrange private health insurance for the members. The retired teachers lost their benefits on retirement, and private insurance companies did not sell health insurance to people over age sixty-five because they were considered high-risk. Andrus contacted Leonard Davis, an insurance broker in New York with Continental Casualty Company, who sold health insurance to groups of retired teachers. Soon Davis was selling health insurance to NRTA members through the mail.

Other retired people who were not teachers also wanted health coverage, leading Andrus and Davis in 1958 to create a nonprofit organization, AARP (the American Association of Retired Persons), to sell health insurance to retired people. (NRTA and AARP officially merged in 1982, though they always functioned as one entity.)[18] Representing AARP in the 1959 hearings before the House Ways and Means Committee, Andrus did not support the Forand Bill. Instead, she proposed a substitute insurance program in which the government would pay premiums to private insurance companies to provide insurance to the elderly.

Davis was an aggressive insurance salesman, and NRTA/AARP membership increased to 750,000 by 1963. When Davis left Continental Casualty in 1965, he bought the company's share of AARP policies and established Colonial Penn.[19] The financial ties between Colonial Penn Insurance and AARP were strong, involving health, life, care, and homeowner insurance policies. Colonial Penn Travel ran AARP's travel service. Mature Temp Services, a Colonial Penn subsidiary, operated employment services for the elderly. At AARP conventions, Colonial Penn products were displayed.

When Andrus died in 1967 at the age of eighty-five, Davis took over leadership of AARP. One year later, he was charged with "untrustworthiness" by the New York State Insurance Commission and lost his insurance license. Although he never admitted to the charge, Davis had several other questionable legal episodes in his career. By the time of his retirement in the early 1980s, Davis's personal net worth was over $160 million.[20]

In the early 1970s, when Bernard Nash became executive director, AARP began to work toward gaining greater influence on government policy.[21] AARP has since grown into a large and influential political organization, dropping the original title and using only its initials; but its activities encompass far more than just politics: it offers members auto insurance, homeowner and life insurance, social events at its four thousand local chapters, a prescription-drug insurance and mail order service, financial services and mutual funds, and travel assistance. Members receive discounts and special offers for airline tickets, auto rentals, ocean cruises, flowers, and hotels. AARP continues to generate about half its revenue from commercial enterprises.[22]

SENIOR CONSCIOUSNESS

In the 1950s and 1960s, both government and private social service organizations began to recognize the importance of senior centers and other formal structures through which seniors could socialize and get professional help and advice. By 1961, a survey by the National Council on Aging found 218 senior citizen centers in existence, each with at least one full-time staff person, along with at least 2,000 senior clubs with no staff.[23] Although the goals of these centers never explicitly included forging a collective political identity, the centers formed a basis for later movements aimed at "senior consciousness."

During the Kennedy administration, although local senior groups existed, they lacked the organization to combine and mobilize on national issues, even those as important as Medicare.[24] In 1961, the White House Conference on Aging offered a bridgehead for a national agenda. The passage of Medicare and the Older Americans Act in 1965 stimulated new interest in and a national awareness of issues affecting elderly citizens. The Older Americans Act established the Administration on Aging, which funds state programs and community organizations that provide services for the elderly. Further, the Age Discrimination Act in 1967 made it illegal to discriminate against people because of age. In 1974, the National Institute of Aging was established to conduct research and training related to the aging process and the diseases and problems of an aging population. White House conferences on aging were repeated in 1971, 1981, and 1995.

Aging organizations founded in the 1970s and 1980s worked mainly to defend the new government programs for the aged. Those organizations that already existed, such as AARP, became more politicized. The new benefits generated a constituency devoted to protecting them. Aging-oriented interest groups grew in number and diversified in mission. Today, older Americans are represented politically by a diverse group of legal and social service organizations with ties to policymakers.

Membership organizations, like the "eight-hundred-pound gorilla" AARP, with its membership of thirty-four million, and smaller groups, such as the Older Women's League (OWL) and the Gray Panthers, exercise political influence through a combination of grassroots organizing and professional and volunteer lobbying. Legal organizations, such as the Center for Medicare Advocacy, the National Senior Citizens Law Center, and California Health Advocates, affect public policy by engaging in class-action lawsuits aimed at forcing Congress to change unfavorable laws or force CMS (formerly HCFA) to enforce Medicare law differently. Some social service organizations working with older Americans, such as the Medicare Rights Center (MRC), influence public policy through congressional testimony and constant communication with appropriate government agencies. Many organizations publish and distribute reports that illustrate the problems experienced by their clients.

Although AARP is more than three times the size of all other aging organizations combined, the aging presence in Washington is diverse.[25] Many organized groups representing the aged, including AARP, are now refurbishing their images and establishing their roles for the future. They consider it essential to capture baby-boomer membership at a time when some politicians are questioning the feasibility of maintaining Medicare and Social Security as entitlement programs for future generations. AARP accepts members as young as fifty and is reshaping its services to focus on this younger group. Whether baby boomers choose to influence policy through organizations or networks that already exist or form new organizations remains to be seen.

THE GRAY LOBBY

The "gray lobby," a nickname for the interest groups representing older Americans, gained considerable respect from lawmakers in the 1980s. Because of the large number of aging organizations, each group tends to carve out its own niche in order to focus its efforts and keep up membership. Many of the most influential organizations focus largely on issues of health policy and are actively involved in the discussion of what the future of Medicare should be.

Activist organizations gain much of their political influence through the sheer numbers of their members, whom elected officials view as valuable voting blocs. Recruitment is crucial for an organization's success. The National Committee to Preserve Social Security and Medicare (NCPSSM), for one, relies heavily on computerized direct-mail campaigns to attract members. Recruitment drives may include material incentives to join, such as discounts and publications.

By mailing in a check for membership, and perhaps occasionally sending a form letter, drafted by the organization, to policy makers, members can make their voices heard with little expense or time commitment. Organizations like the National Council of Senior Citizens (NCSC), Gray Panthers, OWL, and the National Association of Retired Federal Employees (NARFE), encourage their members to join local chapters, which then coordinate efforts to support national causes. AARP's numerous local chapters, by contrast, are social rather than political in nature, and only about 3 percent of AARP's membership actually belongs to one.[26] About 250,000 AARP members are trained as political and service volunteers.

Families USA, established in 1981 to advocate for the elderly poor, has narrowed its focus almost exclusively to health care, especially Medicaid and Medicare; the National Council on Aging has become very involved in health affairs; and OWL is involved in a nationwide Medicare education campaign funded by the Kaiser Family Foundation. AARP's agenda is broad, but the organization has recently focused its political energy on preserving the integrity of Medicare and Social Security, passage of the recent Medicare prescription drug benefit, and now on improving many inadequate provisions of that act.

THE 1990S: A NEW ORDER

By the early 1990s, the favorable attitude toward the gray lobby changed as the public consensus over the necessity and worth of age-related benefits succumbed to ideological conflict. Many conservatives began advocating major reductions in Medicare and Social Security spending. Opposed to government-run entitlement programs, many began to blame older citizens and the interest groups that represented them for consuming a disproportionate percentage of the federal budget with their programs. Some groups framed arguments in terms of "generational equity," asserting that younger Americans are penalized by the greed of the older generation.[27]

In this political environment, at least three conservative aging organizations were formed: the Seniors Coalition, the United Seniors Association (USA), and the 60/Plus Association. These groups joined the National Alliance of Senior Citizens (NASC) in supporting the conservative ideology of limited government involvement in social programs and partial or full support for the privatization of Medicare and Social Security benefits. Beginning between 1989 and 1992 as direct-mail fund-raising organizations, the three groups have since enhanced their research and lobbying capacities. Allied with the Republican "Contract with America" movement in 1994, they lobbied heavily for many of the Medicare budget cuts mandated in BBA 1997.

The existence of conservative as well as traditionally liberal aging organizations attests to the diversity in the political views of older adults, foreshadowing the diversity that can be expected from the baby boomers as well. On the other hand, it is unclear how many older Americans fully support the goals of organizations that want to eliminate Social Security and Medicare as guaranteed benefits. Direct-mail solicitations can be complicated and misleading, and people of all ages contribute.

Public opinion surveys show continued, uniform support for Medicare, but the support weakens when the program is linked with the cost of dramatic tax increases. One survey, for instance, found that more than 60 percent of respondents supported expanding Medicare to cover long-term care, prescription drugs, and younger adults, but only one-third supported raising payroll taxes to pay for these expansions.[28]

AARP LEADERSHIP

Headquartered in Washington, DC, with thirty-four million members, AARP is the second-largest membership organization in the United States; only the Catholic Church is larger. AARP grew quickly after 1965, reaching over six million members in late 1973 and nine million in 1975. By that time, as one of the largest voluntary bodies in the country, it was known for its immense power in national politics.[29] The reputation persists today. In 1997, 1998, and 1999, AARP was ranked by *Fortune* magazine as the lobbying group with "the most clout in Washington" and topped the list of "the Power 25." AARP often leads the old-age lobby in identifying goals and priorities and is a strong supporter of both Medicare and Social Security. In one study, representatives of conservative aging organizations overwhelmingly named AARP as their principal adversary.[30]

Choosing political priorities based on the needs of its membership often translates into AARP's advocating for issues not solely related to aging policy. For instance, AARP was a lead member of the coalition in favor of the Family and Medical Leave Act (FMLA), which, after an eight-year fight, was finally signed into law by President Clinton in 1993.

Although many people think of the FMLA as an act for guaranteeing leave for parents of new babies, AARP and other senior groups expanded the legislation to cover employees who need to take time off from work to care for their parents as well. Under FMLA, employees of medium-sized and large employers can take up to twelve weeks of unpaid leave per year to care for a child, spouse, or parent, or for their own health needs.

AARP devotes substantial resources to educating and mobilizing its members on policy issues. AARP/Vote, begun in 1986, educates and involves older voters on issues of concern to older Americans, and the community at large, at both the state and national levels. Every state has a volunteer AARP/Vote coordinator, who oversees a system of district coordinators—one for each congressional district—supported by teams of district volunteers.[31] The district teams meet regularly with local congressional representatives and other officials.

With such a large membership, AARP cannot always be sure all its members will support its political agenda. One painful conflict occurred between 1988 and 1990, when the organization's support of the Medicare Catastrophic Care Act alienated some of its members and may have damaged its credibility as the political voice for all seniors. The bill offered major improvements to the Medicare benefits package, including coverage for long-term care and prescription drugs. AARP supported the bill, though it risked losing its own lucrative Medigap insurance business. Wealthy seniors opposed it because their premiums would increase for services already covered by their Medigap policies.

Congress passed the Catastrophic Coverage Act amid great concern about government spending deficits. To pay for the new Medicare benefits, Congress instituted an additional premium, to be paid on a sliding scale that protected the less affluent. Although the average senior would pay an increase of only $48 a year, about 6 percent of seniors would have to pay the maximum increase of $800 in the first year, rising to $1,050 in 1993.[32] AARP initially fought to avoid the premium increase by supporting a general tax increase but finally accepted the premium option as a reasonable trade-off for the increased benefits, in part because most of the more affluent would be able to drop their Medigap policies once the new benefits were added to Medicare.

Some groups of elders responded to the premium increase with an intensely negative grassroots reaction. The opposition was vociferous and organized, resulting in a highly publicized episode in which Representative Dan Rostenkowski of Illinois cowered in his car as elderly people threw tomatoes at him. Following the passage of the new law, organizations that opposed it, such as the United Seniors of America and the Conservative Caucus, embarked on a direct-mail campaign urging seniors to make cash donations to repeal the bill.[33] Congress overwhelmingly repealed the Catastrophic Coverage Act just over a year after it was passed.

Another conflict occurred in 1994, when AARP strongly supported President Clinton's Health Security Act, which would have expanded health insurance to working people and families. A small number of AARP members strongly opposed the organization's position, and some dropped their memberships. In 1997, AARP advocated against the BBA cuts in Medicare, which were enacted anyway. A similar controversy occurred in 2003 over the Medicare Modernization Act, which AARP eventually supported. Some of its members saw the act as an expensive payoff to drug companies, yielding a complicated and fundamentally inadequate drug benefit that would not help most seniors. Indeed, AARP itself began lobbying to limit drug prices a week after supporting the legislation that prohibited Medicare from negotiating for lower prices.

AARP has also come under attack from outside. In the early 1990s, it was involved in a controversy over whether it should be permitted to retain its tax-free status despite its extensive retail sales. AARP was engaged in a long dispute with the IRS, and in 1993 it paid $135 million "in lieu of" taxes for the years 1985 through 1993 and added another $15 million in 1994. The organization made a $2.8 million payment to the Post Office in 1993 to settle an accusation over the use of its nonprofit mailing privilege for product solicitations. AARP now uses commercial rates for all its product mailings.

In 1999, AARP settled its fifteen-year fight with the IRS over its tax-exempt status by paying $52 million in back taxes and agreeing to establish a for-profit subsidiary called AARP Services, Inc. During a congressional investigation, Senator Alan Simpson (R-Wyoming), chair of the Social Security and Family Policy Committee and a close friend of the first President Bush, denounced AARP's membership base as "millions of people in search of airline discounts."[34] The president of 60/Plus Association, a conservative senior advocacy group, called AARP "a huge fraud on seniors, profiting by commission from a variety of moneymaking schemes, receiving millions of taxpayer dollars, and promoting programs of big government and high taxes which hurt, not help, seniors."[35]

CNN reported on June 29, 1999, that some politicians were supporting expanding Medicare to include prescription-drug coverage in order to earn the votes of the older Americans in their districts, since older Americans make up a disproportionate share of the voting population.[36]

Interestingly, there is no evidence that AARP has any influence on how older Americans actually vote.[37] Although AARP has thirty-four million members, they do not all vote in support of AARP's political positions. The baby boomers, representing a wide range of social positions and political views, will play a major role in shaping AARP's future. A unified voice may be difficult to achieve.

How Elders Vote

Although senior citizens make up less than 16 percent of the current voting-age population, they constitute about 20 percent of the voters in presidential elections. They are more likely to vote at every election than younger voters. The "gray lobby," led by AARP, has created the perception that older Americans vote as a bloc and will consistently vote against any cuts in Medicare and Social Security. Consequently, these two programs have sometimes been known as the "third rail" of American politics—programs that might kill the career of any politician who touches them.

This assessment may have been accurate as recently as a decade ago, but the situation is now changing. Medicare was subjected to enormous budget cuts with BBA 1997, and many members of Congress wanted to cut further and privatize both Medicare and Social Security. Part of their change in attitude might be due to an enhanced understanding of how today's elders really vote. Demographic polling data show that the elderly do not vote as a bloc. In fact, an analysis of voting patterns of older Americans in presidential elections reveals that citizens sixty-five and over essentially vote with the same variance as younger voters and for the same reasons.[38]

Most studies confirm that age itself has little effect on how people vote. Analyzing many studies of political ideology, Christine Day found that older citizens hold opinions as diverse as those of other age groups on most political issues, including aging policy, with their views affected by race, sex, income, education, occupation, social class, and region.[39] Some evidence suggests that older people have political views not very different from those of younger people. Other polls show that older people are only slightly more concerned than others with aging issues, such as Social Security and Medicare.[40] Today, older citizens are less likely than before to uniformly support government benefits for seniors, and aging baby boomers may reflect even more diverse political positions.

Other factors besides age encourage diverse views that will continue to challenge the efforts of aging interest groups to represent coherent policy directions. Without following groups of people over time to track how their views change with age, we cannot be confident about the significance of age as an independent factor and thus cannot predict the political views of the boomers as they age.

At least one study has found that younger people are actually more supportive of government programs for seniors. The 1998 Americans Discuss Social Security survey found that the 18–29 age group, sometimes called Generation X, showed greater support than any other group for maintaining a safety net for the elderly and for poor children.[41] By more than two to one, this age group favored government intervention to help people avoid poverty in retirement. Those aged sixty-five and older were evenly divided on the same question.

The survey also showed a fairly even division in sentiment among younger people over whose responsibility it is to make sure families have adequate health insurance: half favored personal responsibility, the other half favored government assistance. Moreover, about half of the respondents agreed with a statement that "all people have the right to receive the health care they need, regardless of how much it costs"; while the other half agreed with an alternative statement that "there are limits to what our society can spend even on health care." On this question, income level, party affiliation, and age made a difference. Those with incomes under $40,000 per year were more likely to favor open-ended care, while those earning over $60,000 were more likely to favor limits. The majority of Democrats supported the first option; the majority of Republicans favored the second. With Medicare in mind, it is notable that nearly 60 percent of Generation X favored open-ended care, compared to only 36 percent of respondents aged sixty-five and older.

Whatever the diversity of their political views, baby boomers are not especially active in promoting them: surveys show that they do not vote as often as older people. Compared with the "greatest generation," which grew up in the 1930s and 1940s, baby boomers read newspapers less frequently and are less likely to join churches or civic organizations.[42] Some other findings, however, suggest hope for greater public participation. A study by the Center on Policy Attitudes found that today's older citizens have a lower sense of political efficacy than those under age sixty-five. The center's poll found that 69 percent of those aged sixty-five and over agree that "officials don't care much what people like me think," compared to 57 percent of those aged nineteen to sixty-five. If this is not an aging effect, then the stronger belief by younger groups that their votes matter and that they can make a difference should predict more active voting behavior than is seen among today's seniors.

Many observers see the views of the boomer generation as decisive in the future politics of Medicare. The increase in population of those aged sixty-five and over alone will lead not only to more Medicare beneficiaries with a definite interest in the security of the program but also to more elderly voters. Will a louder chorus of advocacy help to make Medicare more effective? The diversity of opinion among today's elders suggests we should not assume any great unanimity in the views of the next generation. Still, one purpose of this book is to help turn the boomers into an educated constituency capable of understanding the many layers of ideology and special interests involved in health care. They may be able to exert a strong positive influence over the politics that will determine the fate of Medicare and the nation's health security.

The Road to MMA

The budget cuts associated with BBA 1997 were in many cases draconian, making it difficult for some beneficiaries with serious and chronic conditions to get the care they needed.[43] The most dramatic example concerned home care. The Congressional Budget Office (CBO) originally projected reductions in Medicare's budget for home care at $16.2 billion through 2002;[44] but a little over a year later, CBO revised its projection upward, predicting cuts of nearly $48 billion, or nearly three times the original amount.[45] Many service providers went out of business, and the number of persons served and the number of visits per patient swiftly declined, falling in many areas to half their former levels.[46]

BBA also modified Medicare's payment rates for hospitals and established a new prospective-payment scheme for providers, including home health care, SNF, and outpatient hospital services, that had previously been reimbursed on the basis of actual costs.[47] In addition, the bill formalized the PACE program combining Medicare and Medicaid and managed care under the Medicare+Choice program as standard beneficiary options.

BBA established a new agency, the Medicare Payment Advisory Committee (MedPAC), whose sole mission is to advise Congress on issues affecting the Medicare program. MedPAC merged two previous organizations, the Prospective Payment Assessment Commission (ProPAC), which dealt with Part A reimbursement, and the Physician Payment Review Commission (PPRC), which dealt with Part B payments to physicians. The new committee has seventeen members, a full-time executive director, and a staff of about thirty analysts. MedPAC is required to issue two reports to Congress annually, in March and June. MedPAC advises Congress in other ways, too, commenting on proposed regulations and reports to Congress by the secretary of the Department of Health and Human Services, offering testimony, briefing congressional staff, and publishing issue briefs.[48]

Recent changes to Medicare have taken place in a climate of increasing political polarization. The failure of the Bipartisan Commission on Medicare in 1999 can be attributed to deep ideological divisions in the goals of the members of the commission and the constituencies they represented. The urge to radically reform Medicare by eliminating social insurance and creating a free market in health care collided with the urge to protect the fundamental social contract on which Medicare was based. There seemed to be no possible compromise.

In 2003, when Congress passed the Medicare Modernization Act, the polarization of the political environment in Washington had dramatically increased, and the Republican Party controlled all three branches of government. The loss of the bipartisan Medicare constituency that Jonathan Oberlander describes in *The Political Life of Medicare* was demonstrated in a rush to construct a bill that would buy votes and at the same time fulfill ideological agendas. The immediate and ostensible purpose of the bill was to provide a long-needed Medicare prescription-drug benefit. The absence of Medicare coverage for pharmaceuticals had been such a sore point and such an obvious shortcoming for so long that it would be hard for anyone to publicly oppose the bill; thus, a very unlikely set of supporters joined to pass it. The bill emerged at a time when the fate of the elder population was extremely visible, particularly in Florida, where controversy still swirled over the handling of many older people's votes in the 2000 presidential election.

The bill included very inadequate coverage for some medications, for some seniors, and only under certain conditions. It also included extraordinary protections for the pharmaceutical industry, even prohibiting Medicare from negotiating lower prices on behalf of its beneficiaries and thereby allowing the pharmaceutical companies to continue to charge the highest prices to the government. This was one reason for the very high price tag for this bill. The cost was originally estimated at $400 billion, but within a few months of its passage, the Congressional Budget Office acknowledged that even at the time of the debate, the more accurate estimates significantly exceeded $550 billion, and a year later increased projections to almost $800 billion. The legislation was nevertheless passed by a Republican-dominated Congress at a time of enormous federal deficits. Ironically, the most conservative Republicans were among the strongest of the few voices opposing the bill because of its fiscal irresponsibility.

The reformers won by including incentive payments to private plans so that seniors would opt out of traditional Medicare and switch to plans sponsored by insurance companies, as well as more traditional delivery systems. This provision was characterized as giving seniors more choice. Another argument in favor of providing financial incentives to the insurance companies, rather than to the patients, was to strengthen private alternatives that potentially could present more comprehensive managed-care alternatives. The history of Medicare+Choice suggested that most of the industry did not have the experience or capability to deliver good geriatric care; instead, they were shaping insurance products that would offer greater complexity (and also greater confusion) to beneficiaries. While some of the more traditional HMOs offering comprehensive care and doing well under Medicare+Choice, such as Kaiser Permanente, would be strengthened by this bill, it could also lead to a dismantling of the traditional social insurance base of Medicare by adding more financial risks to each patient in this process.

Whatever happens during the implementation of MMA, it is a bill that fails to address the needs for better comprehensive care and the delivery of modern, efficient geriatric medicine. Even AARP, which supported the bill, began a campaign within a week of its passage pointing out all of the bill's defects and calling for numerous changes. Perhaps the reason AARP supported it, as some said, was that they understood what a struggle it is to pass such legislation and thought it was better to work on improving an imperfect bill than miss the opportunity to pass any bill at all.

PLANNING THE FUTURE

Ever since Medicare was founded, Congress has reacted to the program's rising costs, implementing financial reforms that affect the quality of medical care for beneficiaries. Pundits often say that Washington does budget policy, not health policy. Fiscal and political motives predominate. Even the unsuccessful Bipartisan Commission on the Future of Medicare never really addressed the straightforward question, "What kind of health care do beneficiaries need?" The commission also failed to take account of dramatic changes in effective medical practices, geriatric expertise, and the changing health profile of the elderly. Its main concern was to contain costs, because it seemed self-evident that fiscal restraint would be necessary to sustain Medicare in some form in the decades ahead.

Threats of trust-fund bankruptcy and intergenerational tensions have come to overshadow the remarkable achievements of Medicare. Although few, if any, politicians have been bold enough to say outright that they want to dismantle Medicare, some now in Congress hope to rid the program of its traditional social-insurance attributes and propose options like vouchers and means testing instead of universal defined benefits and health security. Such changes would reshape the fundamental values of Medicare. The sea change in the current political arena tests public commitment to a social contract for health care. The next chapter looks more closely at this commitment in order to clarify what we expect Medicare to achieve and how to accomplish it.

Ideally, we should start from scratch and build a new Medicare program that reflects both modern health-care knowledge and the needs of the modern aging society, and then adopt payment structures to make it affordable. But Congress, surrounded by political pressure and industry lobbyists, determines what kind of medical care older Americans can afford in an unsystematic and haphazard way. Producing a few good results in specific areas does not address fundamental problems. Moreover, incremental legislation lacks a vision of coordinated care. Instead, rules fit together poorly, contradict one another, and appear irrational.

One of the current criticisms of Medicare, and of modern American medical practice in general, is that there is too much focus on expensive treatments and not enough attention to prevention strategies that could actually reduce costs. Today, medical specialty interest groups can be as influential as the AMA and often disagree with the AMA's policy positions, lobbying to protect Medicare payments for their own special services. Such divisions within the community of physicians have added to the fragmentation of Medicare's benefits. No one is advocating for a comprehensive, patient-oriented insurance model.

Clearly, in today's rapidly changing health-care environment, physicians and families need increased flexibility to provide each person with the right mix of care and services. Patients need the ability to choose treatment options based on their values and prognoses, without the perverse incentives, obstacles, and gaps induced by Medicare payment policies. Elected officials bear the responsibility to decide the extent to which the system should be publicly funded. These are ethical and ideological questions that are difficult in the abstract and become even more challenging when the answers involve real money and the health of real people and are being argued by diverse and powerful interest groups in the arena of national politics.

CHAPTER 11

Rationing Is Inevitable

As early as 1959, a Congressional study addressed the "revolution of rising expectations" in health care and questioned the current system's ability to finance it in the future.[1] Even then, policy makers were concerned about rising costs, as the abilities of medical science expanded and health care became a significant portion of the national economy. Between 1928 and 1961, health-care spending increased by about 700 percent, rising from 3.6 percent to 5.7 percent of GNP. By 1990 it had increased to 12 percent, and by 2004 it exceeded 14 percent of GNP—significantly more than in any other nation.[2]

Some experts project health spending will grow 2 or 3 percent a year over the next seventy-five years, mostly driven by the cost of new medical technologies.[3] Under this assumption, health spending would eventually account for 30 percent of GDP. Although it is impossible to accurately predict spending trends seventy-five years into the future, there is no denying that paying for modern medical technologies is a serious challenge. The Medicare Part A trust fund that pays for hospital benefits is currently projected to run out of money some time between 2021 and 2025.

Historian Rosemary Stevens observes, "Medicare was designed to be responsive to the technological and high-cost side of medicine, rather than to chronic illness. Paramount concerns in the early 1960s were the financial needs of the expanding hospital system and the pocketbook needs of the retired population."[4] In other words, income security rather than health security was the goal. A primary question in Medicare reform today should be whether this mission remains acceptable. To achieve high-quality care, modern geriatric medicine requires that patients and their families make health care decisions based on medical science and careful personal choice, not on what Medicare pays. To ensure health security without going broke will require setting limits—both on *how much* Medicare pays and on *what* Medicare pays for. Ideally, this would be done based on scientific evidence and geriatric expertise, rather than on lobbying battles. But such a "rational" approach will have to involve rationing.

Price Allocation

To cope with increasing costs, Medicare and other insurance programs have rationed benefits by strictly limiting the range of coverage. Growing expressions of indignation over coverage gaps for the insured, and over the complete lack of coverage for one-seventh of the population, indicate that this form of health care rationing is increasingly unacceptable to the public. Although universal coverage is supposed to eliminate problems with continuity of care and price barriers, it will surely not remove price rationing completely. Cost containment is a prerequisite for expanded coverage, and price is a necessary aspect of containing the demand for services. Beneficiary cost sharing through deductibles and co-payments is a legitimate way of limiting utilization of desirable benefits, so long as out-of-pocket expenses do not become a barrier to needed care.

Ideas for Medicare reform that expand benefits but impose large deductibles represent a conscious decision to reintroduce price rationing in the allocation of health care. Among the many problems with such ideas is the fact that few people have the knowledge, access to information, cognitive capacity, or motivation to be prudent purchasers of health care. Some Medicare reformers propose expanding benefits but imposing large deductibles, in the hope of encouraging patients to become more price-conscious in deciding whether to undergo expensive treatments or services.[5] Further, as many observers point out, individuals are largely unable or unwilling to accurately assess future risks and expenses.

Faith in abstract market principles has also put other forms of price rationing on the agenda for health-care reform, such as proposals for medical savings accounts. Such notions represent more than an impractical application of market ideology. They imply that we are uncomfortable about making explicit rationing decisions in a public manner, especially in regard to a vital good like health care. No one wants to be held responsible for avoidable suffering or death. Price rationing transfers the responsibility back to the individual. Decisions about restricting services are not seen as being imposed from above by insurers or the government: in theory, people are making their own decisions in a sphere where there is no moral role for the rest of society. We need to revisit the issue of moral responsibility and the reasons for employing social insurance in the first place.

Implicit Allocation

Medical practitioners are always making decisions about when and how to provide care—and, by implication, when to withhold it. Although there is merit in allowing flexibility for implicit rationing, that is, rationing care at the physician's discretion (which is bound to persist in any system to some degree), practitioners usually tend to use all available treatment resources to maximize efficacy. As a result, expensive treatments are rarely forgone, so long as payment arrives. From the physician's point of view, explicit decisions to ration resources are based mostly on the chances of success: a physician may refrain from suggesting treatments she judges unlikely to improve the outcome for an individual patient.[6] Cost consciousness has been, for the most part, outside the practitioner's domain, and perhaps rightly so. But if that is the case, cost control must be instituted by another means.

This picture of ideal clinical judgment, with medical resources fairly distributed according to need, is not always the reality. Studies in both the United Kingdom and United States indicate that physicians regularly deny treatment on the basis of age and other social factors.[7] In a recent national survey in the United States, physicians believed that unfair treatment is mostly based on whether patients have health insurance, followed by how well they speak English, their level of education, and their financial status.[8] Such social prejudices would be hard to justify aloud. This form of implicit rationing has no legitimacy. One goal of quality improvement is to make these implicit decisions more explicit by including and informing patients about treatment options.

Relying on implicit rationing may also burden physicians and other providers with extremely difficult ethical decisions. A physician who is expected both to do his utmost to heal a patient and to keep costs down is confronted with a role conflict. In the United Kingdom, physicians are expressing resentment that they are expected to assume both roles due to the imposition of financial risk that results from their having to manage their patients within a budget.[9] This dual role poses a real tension between the physician's public trust and responsibility toward the patient.

On the one hand, given the need to set limits on the costs of care, if the physician acts only as the patient's advocate, then limits will have to be set by external forces. Insurers or the government will specify the scope of coverage and refuse to pay for certain goods and services. In this situation, physicians tend to become frustrated because their professional judgment about individual patients' needs is constrained by external restrictions; but at least the physician and patient are on the same team.

On the other hand, if the physician is involved in setting limits, the patient's trust may be lost, as happened in the backlash against HMOs during the 1990s. Patient complaints, supported by numerous court decisions, produced a clear message that rewarding physicians too much for restricting patient care is unacceptable.

Yet equitable rationing decisions require medical knowledge. Health professionals have the clinical knowledge on which to base allocation decisions, and their immediate experience with patients' needs enables them to personalize care much more responsibly than an external administrator could. If allocation decisions must be made, a trusted clinician may be the person best qualified to make them. The physician can also be assisted by standards of evidence-based practice or cost efficiency supplied by expert analysis. In particularly difficult ethical dilemmas—when resources are scarce, as with organ transplants, or in deciding the terms of treatment near the end of life—then community standards, reviewed protocols, hospital rules, and legal requirements can provide guidance and help physicians, patients, and families accept the consequences of the decisions they make. The most important aspect of the decision-making process is transparency, with an established system of accountability and procedures for input and dialogue.

Rational Allocation

Obviously, before explicit decisions are made to ration or withhold care, those responsible must make every effort to maximize resources by eliminating waste and ensure equity by reducing variability in the system. This was the goal of managed care in the 1990s. Notable progress was made in some areas, but a sense of distrust developed when the public perceived that profits, rather than better care, were often the motive. Activism is growing for radical quality improvement, on the principle that evidence and science, embedded in organized management systems, can reduce unnecessary costs and improve health outcomes.[10] One central goal of quality improvement involves information systems and decision tools.

Prescribing drugs is one area where information technology can definitely help to control costs and avoid adverse events. Computerizing patient records, including a history of prescriptions filled, allows the physician to review how the current prescription fits with others. An interactive system that prompts for adverse reactions would greatly reduce harm, particularly among elderly patients who frequently take multiple medications. A system allowing physicians to transmit prescriptions directly to pharmacies would reduce additional errors due to misinterpretation of handwritten slips.

A second goal in this area is to maximize value through prudent purchasing. An electronic information system facilitates the employment of drug formularies, which are gaining acceptance (over stiff resistance from the pharmaceutical industry) as a means of comparing drugs according to cost-effectiveness. International collaboration is under way to share data from the clinical trials that are the basis of the formularies.[11] The recently evolved methodology of research synthesis provides a more reliable and hence convincing bias for rationing decisions than has heretofore been available. Multiple clinical trials addressing a single issue are combined statistically in a "systematic review" to produce the balance of evidence. Systematic reviews can assist policy makers to ration effectively if analyses of cost-effectiveness are made in a way that permits broad public discussion of the values input by the economists doing the analysis. The National Institution for Clinical Evaluation (NICE) in the UK has recently shown the way forward on this, as has the Drug Evaluation Review Project, a collaborative enterprise by fifteen states, Canada, and the large California Public Employees' Retirement System (CalPERS).

A prescription drug formulary is one of several promising initiatives for evidence-based practice using electronic information systems to organize complex information and integrate it at the point of service. Evidence-based systems can also provide decision tools that allow providers and patients together to review options and risks in detail.[12] Although this approach is sometimes criticized as "cookbook medicine," individual characteristics necessarily leave plenty of room for professional judgment to operate, much as a good recipe allows for variation while providing a clear and tested (evidence-based) protocol.

Victor Fuchs and Alan M. Garber advocate the extension of evidence-based practice into the realm of medical technology, funding a national center to conduct research and disseminate systematic information.[13]

There are endless new (and costly) medical technologies being developed, but some contribute to health much more than others. Increasing and organizing information favors cost control and quality improvement by promoting better decisions, prudent purchasing, and patient understanding of these choices.

Disease-management programs are another avenue for reducing costs and improving quality of care and are used increasingly by managed-care plans and others. Independent firms often offer these services under contract and promise significant savings. Management of chronic conditions is itself expensive, and cost savings in some cases are minor; but reduction of avoidable complications and quality improvement have been demonstrated.

One disincentive to such programs is that in fee-for-service health-care systems, the insurance company realizes the savings, while doctors and hospitals make less money. Another drawback is that although older people often have more than one chronic disease (for instance hypertension, diabetes, and heart failure often occur together), most disease-management programs focus only on a single condition. Often, indeed, the programs are supported by a pharmaceutical company with a product that treats a specific condition seeking a market in just that area.[14] In contrast, geriatric medicine aims for the comprehensive management of multiple chronic conditions and an orientation to the needs of the person, not just the disease. The right approach to setting limits for Medicare spending must take the principles of geriatric medicine into account.

Resource Allocation

Countries with universal health-care systems have to rely on resource rationing in order to provide affordable coverage for everyone. Citizens in these countries must sometimes cope with long waiting lists for treatment; such lists are one means of prioritizing urgent needs and maintaining equity. In the United States, the terrors of waiting lists have been exaggerated by opponents of systematic universal coverage; they disregard the fact that in the current health-care system in this country, those with no insurance coverage cannot get even basic treatment. We are currently spending so much more on health care than any other country that we should be able to prioritize care without resorting to months-long waiting lists. With adequate funding and a rational allocation of resources, no one needs to be excluded or their treatment unreasonably delayed.

We can provide timely, equitable coverage if we save money in other ways, and one clear way to do this is to limit expensive treatments that have a limited chance of success. Currently, Medicare pays for many very expensive treatments with unpromising outcomes. We apparently have no political will for the controversial task of rational resource allocation. Experience elsewhere also suggests that we could have comparable outcomes with appropriate supervision of waiting lists. Making rationing explicit would allow us to give priority to treatments that are urgent and those that are known to be effective.

Experience with organ transplants has provided valuable experience with resource allocation. Published protocols by specialty societies and UNOS (the United Network for Organ Sharing) help guide U.S. processes of rationing. Similar practices are used in other countries. Three decision rules are commonly used for fairly establishing priority for waiting lists: severity of the condition; time on the waiting list; and, when order or outcome is unclear, random selection.

A committee in western Canada developing standards for waiting lists for elective care has made a useful distinction between severity and urgency.[15] *Urgency* is reserved to evaluate the likelihood of different outcomes. A condition can be severe but not expected to deteriorate. Patients with a condition not yet judged overly severe can be moved up on the list by the expectation of deterioration if treatment is delayed or a much better prospect of recovery. The two terms together appear to help ensure a fair distribution of resources.[16] A related distinction is observed in international guidelines for lung transplants, endorsed in the United States, where urgency is included as contraindication.[17] Conditions susceptible to poorer outcomes are given a lower priority.

Another form of health-care rationing is the Oregon Plan, almost defunct now but recognized as a means of prioritizing and standardizing diagnosis and treatment. Treatment decisions were partly based on a prioritized list, established by the State of Oregon for its Medicaid program, that paired diagnosis and treatment and then ranked the pairs by associated benefit and cost. A dozen additional community values solicited from stakeholders and focus groups were used to make small adjustments in the priorities. Extensive dialogue with residents throughout the state ensured support for the list. The original intention was to ration resources explicitly in order to expand Medicaid to cover more uninsured people, including working families below the poverty level. State and federal budget cuts in recent years have limited Oregon's ability to expand coverage as much as originally hoped, but the plan did instill a basis for explicit and evidence-based rationing.

Traditional Medicaid is like Medicare in that it provides specific benefits; but since it is not a universal-entitlement program like Medicare, states typically adjust it to their budgets by limiting eligibility. Consequently, some people get extensive benefits, and others get nothing. The Oregon Health Plan devised a rational way to limit benefits in order to offer insurance to as many people as possible.

The Oregon Plan provides a "menu" for effective medical treatment, somewhat analogous to a drug formulary. It provides a rational basis for determining medical necessity. A treatment very likely to extend life would receive priority over a treatment that has only a slim chance of success. The widespread respect for the list is evidently due to the public process by which it was created as well as the proof that devising such a list is possible. As a lesson for any rationing proposal, the Oregon Plan highlights the value of open dialogue to legitimize such critical decisions.

A singular effort to manage the allocation of resources in the United States is represented by state certificate-of-need (CON) programs, designed to regulate hospital investments and limit the spread of medical technology. CON, mandated by federal law between 1974 and 1986, is still operating in many states. A state agency must approve construction of new medical facilities. The regulation is generally unpopular, apparently only minimally effective, and often trumped by political pressures. New hospitals and imaging centers are usually approved even if not really necessary. Enforcement appears to be unenthusiastic in many states and operates without a clear guiding principle. Apparently, regulation is neither effective nor well-accepted without a corresponding vision of its purpose.

Health-care rationing in the United States is mainly effected by lack of insurance coverage. As a result, we have no explicit or widely accepted way to curb expenditures, and the fragmented system hinders us from doing so. Few people in authority are able to concentrate on the public good as a whole in the health-care system. The competitive marketplace is not intended or designed to further the public good. Insurance companies reduce payments to doctors and hospitals, "carve out" benefits—like pregnancy and delivery, or mental health—or add high copayments and deductibles to shift costs to patients. Medicare follows the private-insurance model in this way, as it has in so many other ways. Pockets of self-interest compete for profit and shift burdens back and forth without achieving any improvement in quality or value of care.

Technology innovation in health care may lead to expensive and unnecessary services, but deciding how to reduce availability is not easy. Escalating health care costs could be justified, even at a rate far greater than the growth of the economy, if the value added by those costs were proportionate. At some point, however, the marginal benefits of innovation will clearly exceed what we are willing to pay. Yet public support for innovation is enormous. Will shifting the cost burden more to patients make them more cautious consumers of technology? Many studies already show that poor people have less access to high-tech forms of care.[18] The public and private investment in technology innovation (and drug research in particular) easily overwhelms narrow local rules attempting to manage resources. Allocation of resources seems the only alternative to a dramatic inequity in access to new medical treatments, further exacerbating disparities in health outcomes between rich and poor.

AGE-BASED ALLOCATION

The types of rationing discussed so far—eliminating waste, reducing the use of less effective measures, and making cost-effective choices of treatments and drugs—are relatively painless for the consumer. If we must go further in curbing costs, we may end up denying care and allowing avoidable adverse events. Some analysts, for example, support age-based rationing of life-sustaining health care.[19] Since there are indications that such rationing already occurs implicitly, it is worth addressing this issue openly in order to reach an explicit consensus that could help overcome prejudices and promote fair clinical decisions.

Clarification of the issues involved in age-based rationing is especially important for Medicare. Some critics of Medicare argue that it is unjust to spend so much on the elderly when children and young people remain uninsured. Although justice across generations is not irrelevant, we also need to be reminded of justice in the context of families. Elderly people are likely to need more medical care, and if Medicare did not exist, families would have to pay, taking those resources away from the younger family members.

Critics also argue that much of what is spent on older people, particularly in the last year of life, is wasted. In terms of cost-effectiveness, however, older patients benefit greatly from early detection of chronic illness and prevention of functional decline through prospective care. Modern medicine offers strategies to help people age successfully into their eighties and nineties. Moreover, the finding that most expenditures occur in the last months or year of life is not affected by age per se. End-of-life care is expensive for everyone, regardless of age. More to the point in this respect, resources expended at the end of life need to be redirected to promote high-quality, appropriate palliative care, which also has its costs. Withholding aggressive treatment could result in some small cost savings. The only problem here is that thus far we have been unable to develop a robust model to pay for clearly effective but low-tech services.

Developing a clear strategy for allocating resources under Medicare would achieve no good purpose if chronological age is used as a decisive factor. The criteria should be health, functional status, and the chances of successful treatment. Age should be only infrequently regarded by physicians as an independent risk factor, and then only in combination with other serious conditions, when it may tip the balance of assessed risk for a treatment strategy.[20]

A final, strong argument against age-based rationing is simply that length of life and quality of life are not comparable.[21] A "fair innings" argument, suggesting that the elderly have had their day and should accept debility and death without complaint, takes no account of individual personality, social and civic engagement, capacity for pleasure and achievement, and so much more that might be added together to assess the value of the years of life remaining to any individual. These factors are not necessarily reduced by old age and may, indeed, be magnified. In rationing care on such a basis, physicians and other health-care practitioners would be obliged to ask their patients, "Who are you?" Emergency personnel would ask, "Why should we save you?" This is clearly contrary to the long tradition of professional ethics in medicine, which rests on beneficence and nonmalfeasance and not on some calculation of the patient's inherent moral or social worth.

Rationing is inevitable. It could be done in many ways that would be deleterious to our social fabric and to our intergenerational communities and families. The best approach is based on the understanding of a framework of social contract and an acceptance of basic health care as a component of that contract.

CHAPTER 12

The Social Contract

Health care in the United States is in chaos. Experts have been exploring and documenting the financing and delivery of health care without managing to develop a comprehensive policy that works. The health-care system, such as it is, perpetuates inefficiency and hardship because of its rapidly escalating costs, lack of insurance coverage, and inadequate quality of care. While medical science continues to advance, we are far from a rational system that allows everyone to benefit.

We live in an era of unprecedented longevity and productive old age. Modern medicine allows us to manage chronic conditions while maintaining high levels of function and quality of life. Yet current patterns of thinking and behavior will not permit our society to flourish in the next century. Very soon we will need to choose: will the aging of society be a great success story leading to increased productivity, health, and respect for older citizens, or will it turn into a crippling burden that devours resources and drives a wedge between young and old?

Successful strategies for responding to these challenges will not emerge from the stark political dichotomies of Democrat or Republican, liberal or conservative. We are all included in the social contract that makes our nation rich and strong. All families benefit when they can protect themselves against financial ruin by spreading the risk of health-care costs across a large population. Together we need to agree on the nature of the social contract and commit ourselves to its implementation.

Foundations of Health Security

In 1935, widespread poverty among the elderly, affecting whole families, compelled the federal government to pass a bill for social security. During the Depression, the elderly were hit even harder than most. By 1934, more than half of the elderly in America lacked sufficient income to support themselves.[1] The resolution that emerged to provide an "escape from misery" was only partial and admittedly inadequate, and it omitted the plans for government-organized health insurance that had been given the most attention at the time.[2] The debates were strongly colored by the ethic of individual responsibility and an intense fervor for profit and an unregulated market, both viewed by many as distinctively American virtues.

Medicare and Medicaid were enacted into federal law in 1965 in response to the stubborn fact that misery persisted among vulnerable populations even when the nation was prospering as never before. Healthcare costs were a growing threat to family stability. In 1964, Lyndon Johnson was elected to the presidency with 61 percent of the vote. Much of his support came from working-age Americans who realized that they would have to subsidize their parents' health care unless Medicare became law. These Americans created an intergenerational social contract because they had a strong incentive to do so. They were also in the midst of what was, until the 1990s, the longest period of economic expansion in American history. They knew how they wanted to spend their increasing disposable income, and it wasn't on their mothers' health care.[3]

Medicare was, and is, a social contract firmly grounded in self-interest. Health care was a clear next step in the evolution of social insurance, following workers' compensation, which was established in most states by 1920, and state unemployment insurance, which was established by 1937. The Social Security pension plan initiated payroll contributions in 1937 and began paying out in 1942. At the same time, federal legislation established grants to states to support needy mothers, children, and other vulnerable persons. Survivor benefits were added to Social Security in 1939. Coverage was extended to previously excluded workers and the self-employed in the 1950s, and disability insurance was added.

Although states and local governments have traditionally been responsible for social welfare, their programs have not always been consistent or reliable. Tax competition is one problem. If tax rates vary among neighboring regions, the areas with lower taxes will draw business enterprises from the others, even though the added services that accompany higher taxes can be advantageous for business. Another long-standing problem is population mobility. Displacement by frontier wars and immigration streams in the eighteenth century burdened local governments with impoverished refugees, who were quickly labeled as vagrants and placed outside the scope of community responsibility.[4] A sensible solution was to move welfare arrangements to a higher level of government, initially the states. In the nineteenth century, as immigration increased, the national government increasingly came to be seen as the appropriate level for comprehensive social programs accommodating a mobile population. National arrangements for social insurance were unthinkable, however, before the federal income tax was established in 1913. By the 1960s, there were plenty of reasons to believe that a national program for health insurance was more likely to succeed than state programs.

By 1934, most states had pension plans of some kind, but they accomplished very little. The average benefit was about 65 cents a day, and eligibility criteria were so restrictive that most poor seniors did not qualify.[5] Only about 3 percent of the elderly received benefits under the state plans. Many older Americans did not even apply for the programs, despite their grave financial situations, because of the stigma associated with financial assistance.

Although the government at all levels was inexperienced with social insurance forty years ago, it would be a mistake to look only this far when evaluating the U.S. experience with the social contract. The federal government already played an important role in creating a uniform and fair environment for the conduct of business. President Franklin Roosevelt recognized the broader context for social insurance in a 1938 speech on Social Security, pointing out that government had served to guarantee the welfare of the rich and the strong, and now rightly moved to meet its obligations to the less fortunate.[6] His point is well illustrated in the history of westward expansion. Speculators and businessmen in new territories were typically eager to gain the protection of the federal government for property rights and the enforcement of private contracts.[7] Guaranteeing fair practices was a later development, first in railroad regulation, then in business markets, banking, and securities.

In addition to overseeing property and capital relations, the social contract also guarantees the rights and relations of employers and labor. Here, the social contract enhances legitimacy and promotes productive, respectful relationships. Mitigating the harsher elements of compulsion in employment allows workers greater autonomy and security and improves productive capacity. This lesson took a long time to learn.

Following the volatile decades of labor unrest during the latter part of the nineteenth century, a number of industry initiatives and federal regulations improved conditions for workers. Progressive legislation led to the creation of the federal Department of Labor in 1913. During this period, private, employer-based welfare programs were consciously designed to "save capitalism."[8] Still, workers in many sectors of the economy lacked basic guarantees of safety and security. Fears of revolution remained potent through the 1930s and peaked in the anticommunist crusade of the 1940s and 1950s.[9]

In this environment, laws respecting the social contract in labor affairs nevertheless secured a basic level of justice and peace. The revolutionary position of labor activists noticeably softened after 1935, once union activities were given official recognition, and mechanisms were established for grievances and arbitration through the National Labor Relations Board.

Partly as a result of this legacy, any government program labeled "social," such as social insurance, acquired an association with socialism. The Red Scare was based on fears of certain conditions inimical to business interests; but many reasonable forms of social, financial, and political organization—like insurance—were also unreasonably branded by opponents as elements of socialism. Thus, Medicare was branded by its opponents as socialized medicine, and great efforts were necessary to overcome this objection.

The traditional social contract also includes basic public goods like the military, police and fire protection, utilities, municipal services, and public health agencies. There is a consensus that such services are necessary and are appropriately administered by government. More controversially, education also has become part of the social contract. Public sponsorship of schooling was firmly resisted until the period between 1870 and 1918, when states overcame the arguments for private responsibility and established minimum attendance laws, supported by tax levies. The value of an educated citizenry for a vibrant, democratic society and a productive workforce finally became too clear to ignore.

The examples here illustrate many features of civil society that are poorly or inefficiently provided by private initiative. Some goods and services, such as highways or police protection, require government intervention to ensure equitable contributions toward a good that benefits everyone. Other goods, like sewage management or airline safety, could perhaps be managed like a private good; but we are not willing to tolerate lapses that could jeopardize lives. Efficiency is also an issue. Why do we abide by road signs and the convention of driving on the right? The social contract of the road goes beyond safety. We recognize that a common investment and established rules of conduct get us where we want to go faster than if we allowed a multiplicity of arbitrary private interests to act entirely independently.

Individualistic and libertarian dissent is often voiced, but enormous majorities support public administration of certain contract relations and conventions. Citizens have sought to raise trust, security, confidence, and predictability to assure the fruits of enterprise, promote efficiency, establish justice, and support freedom. Basic security is essential for all kinds of business practice, for personal liberties, and for the prosperity of the whole nation. A foundation of shared investment and shared benefit for the fortunate and the unfortunate alike helps us all.

Moral Responsibility for Health

Social insurance, and particularly social health insurance, is a relatively new aspect of the social contract, and one born of crisis. Health problems and substantial medical debt are primary factors in personal bankruptcies in the United States, along with job loss and family problems, which are also frequently related to health.[10] Over 40 percent of all bankruptcies in 1999 were associated with a medical condition or debt. Half of those in bankruptcy had health insurance, indicating that coverage is frequently inadequate. Nearly half of the bankruptcies among those aged sixty-five and over were due to a medical reason.

A market economy, as promoted in the United States, tends to view medical expenses as just another form of personal consumption and to disapprove of collective or government action to reduce insecurity. In contrast, in free-market European countries with universal health systems, individual bankruptcy due to health costs is unthinkable. Although many countries encounter problems in providing high-quality, well-coordinated health-care services, the United States is unique in the anxiety its citizens experience over health-care costs.[11]

Why this should remain so is a mystery. In spite of the political rhetoric, public opinion polls show that most people (66 percent) would prefer the government to provide needed services rather than cut taxes; nearly half (44 percent) prefer more services with higher taxes; and a large majority (80 percent) would prefer to maintain spending levels on education, health care, and Social Security than to lower taxes. Social Security is by far the most popular tax, with very few (9 percent) disliking it.[12]

An exploration of public opinion in Germany yields similar results.[13]

In spite of financial difficulties and criticism by market-oriented theorists, the system of universal health insurance maintains strong public support. In the public perception, four principles of solidarity for social health insurance stand out:

1. Health risks are regarded as more or less ruled by chance and only slightly influenced by personal behavior;

2. For health, providing benefits according to need is seen as preferable to providing benefits according to ability to pay;

3. Personal interest is satisfied by an assurance of reciprocity;

4. The costs of severe disease are seen as too heavy to bear alone.

These principles support a relationship of trust between the individual and society. The system is regarded as fair. Economic theory recognizes that market behavior is commonly influenced by a sense of fairness and not by self-interest alone.[14] The idea of "fairness" influencing behavior is supported by studies in behavioral game theory.[15] A perception of fair behavior elicits favor, while a perception of unfair behavior elicits resistance even at the expense of self-interest. Part of the problem in achieving solidarity in the United States is a lack of trust in the national government, with 52 percent of the population trusting the government only some of the time, and an additional 12 percent trusting it none of the time.[16]

Thousands of pages of scholarly treatises in political theory and bioethics attest to our ambivalence on the issue of social solidarity in health care. Actually, the word *ambivalence* may grant too much credit to our existing policies, which instead display a murky confusion.

For example, how do we reconcile our seemingly contradictory beliefs that everyone should have access to some kind of health insurance, but we all must exercise individual choice and responsibility? If a critically ill person is brought by ambulance to an emergency room in a public hospital, we consider it unethical (and illegal) not to provide whatever life-saving care is possible, even if the person is uninsured or incapable of paying. Private hospitals are held to this standard by federal regulations. Other safety-net programs demonstrate that we are equally unwilling to refuse necessary health-care services to those who need them, even if they are directly responsible for causing their own medical problems. Apparently, we do believe in some kind of right to health care.

Although the United States ostensibly operates a private market for health care, federal and state governments fund community health care for the uninsured. In 2001 they reimbursed providers about $31 billion for uncompensated care.[17] Private philanthropy and a "cost shift" to private payers covers an additional few billion dollars' worth of care for those unable to pay. A large portion of care for the uninsured is paid through special formulas in Medicare and Medicaid reimbursement. Many physicians follow a long-standing practice of forgiving debts for those with lower incomes or struck by misfortune who cannot afford to pay for services. It seems odd to insist on market principles in health care when we are obviously unwilling to accept the consequences. Indeed, a market will not work effectively under such circumstances.

Whether health care is a right is not simply a philosophical question. There are practical consequences to consider. If an indigent person is not turned away, who pays for the treatment? Are we paying for it in the most efficient manner? Does it make sense to allow uncertainty and poor health to prevail, only to step in late in the process and likely pay higher costs? Is it fair to shift money from insured patients to create a safety net for the uninsured? Should we provide the uninsured with early detection and preventive care that will lessen human and financial costs from serious illness down the road? If we care about both cost savings and humanitarian issues, then what policies would reflect this caring?

Modern medicine, with its increasing awareness of the benefits of prevention and chronic-disease management, has made this issue more salient. We know that careful control of diabetes, for example, reduces the predictable complications of the disease. The consequences of inattention can be serious, including heart attacks, kidney failure, blindness, and peripheral vascular damage that can lead to amputation. Diabetes is common among the elderly and becoming more prevalent among those under sixty-five. A young uninsured man with diabetes is unlikely to get primary care to help manage his condition, particularly the intensive type that prevents complications. If he has a heart attack or develops gangrene of a leg and goes to an emergency room, he is treated for the acute problem; but the facility has no legal responsibility to provide ongoing management for his chronic illness. Unless he is lucky enough to connect with a charity program, once out of the hospital the patient is basically on his own again. Ironically, if his kidneys fail as a consequence of his diabetes, Medicare will step in to pay for dialysis and all his medical care, even that unrelated to the kidney disease.

This example can be multiplied by millions. Taking responsibility for one's own health is extremely important and needs to be promoted, along with greater responsibility for a clean and safe physical environment and a social environment that encourages healthy activities; but certain circumstances also require medical management that is safe, effective, efficient, and timely, for which individuals need assistance. We know we can do better, and we should.

In 1983, a presidential commission published a report, *Securing Access to Health Care*,[18] which argued forcefully that universal health-care coverage should be considered a moral responsibility and supported by the public and by government action. The commission refused to call health care a right, as many other nations have done. With escalating health-care costs devouring budgets, such caution may be appropriate. Calling it a moral responsibility rather than a right allows a measure of flexibility: what level of morality can we afford? The implication here is that establishing a right to health care implies a corollary responsibility, and our society has not been willing to assign that responsibility to anyone. Policy debates over the last decade indicate that we do not want government to do it all; neither are we willing to rely on employers or individuals alone. The notion of a "right" will remain theoretical until we clearly assign the obligation to select and purchase health care.

To justify its argument for moral responsibility, the commission emphasized the role of chance, claiming that individuals suffer ill-health through no fault of their own. This is largely true; but we know, of course, that healthy or unhealthy behaviors can make a considerable difference in risk factors. The commission did not address this issue, leaving unanswered the question of whether our moral responsibility should extend only to those who deserve it. This is, after all, the very term by which we tend to negotiate income support, stipulating that assistance should go only to the "deserving" poor. The commercial insurance market is adept at making such distinctions of risk and pricing policies by experience rating. High risks are either excluded or face prohibitive premiums, penalizing people for health conditions over which they have no control. Should we make similar distinctions in a public program for health care?

Different groups of people answer this question in different ways. The professional responsibility of a physician is to treat the patient, regardless of the irresponsible behavior that brings a person to the emergency room or clinic. Research in various countries indicates that physicians favor equitable treatment for everyone foremost, and would prefer to lobby for more resources rather than deny appropriate care.[19] On the other hand, the public tends to feel that people who smoke or suffer sports injuries should be held partly accountable. The sense of moral responsibility diminishes with the element of chance involved in the health risk.

Guaranteed health-care coverage might encourage risky behavior by assuring that care will be available if needed, but how we would make distinctions of accountability is a problem. We may not want to discourage some risky behaviors, like participation in sports or certain useful but risky occupations, like firefighting or commercial fishing. Other behaviors, like poor nutrition and obesity, could be extremely difficult to categorize as a matter of personal or public responsibility. Levels of physical and mental exercise, which make a significant difference to health, would be impossible to measure or monitor. In yet other cases, like smoking, the average risk rate will not capture individual differences; genetic susceptibility and environment make identical behavior more or less risky for each person.

In general, the process of distinguishing accountability, if done fairly, could become an endless and infinitely complex task bound to invite arbitrary decisions, conflict, and inefficiency. A simpler and more equitable solution is to accept a moral responsibility for health care for all, and work separately to promote safety and healthy behaviors.

In the United States the idea of no-fault insurance began in the 1970s with auto insurance. Despite adoption by several states and signs of success, the approach remains highly controversial, with tort lawyers naturally opposing the idea and issues of consumer choice and options for tort remedies in extreme cases forming a thicket of arguments not easily resolved.[20] Among the chief points of contention is the argument that if no-fault insurance encourages risky behaviors, then some other incentive must be established to avoid overuse of benefits, otherwise the system will eventually be bankrupted. For health care, this contention points to health promotion as a necessary part of the system. Extending the argument for no-fault insurance, the administration of workers' compensation could be greatly simplified by eliminating experience rating on business premiums. Health and safety goals might be better pursued separately.[21] Some argue that the no-fault idea should also be implemented in medical tort reform. Again, incentives and assurance for safety might be instituted separately.

Even without overuse of benefits, the high cost of new drugs and technologies, if unrestricted, is bound to bring such a system to a tipping point. A sense of moral responsibility might lead us to decide that we can afford everything for everyone; but that would require giving up other goods and services, which in turn would reduce our general prosperity. More likely we will find that in defining our moral responsibility for providing health care, we will need to consider setting limits; and here we return to the ever-present debate over health-care rationing.

The Medicare Contract

One of the greatest advantages of a large, mandatory government insurance program like Medicare is its ability to spread risk across a large population and over time. The strength of the Medicare contract lies in its inclusivity and stability. Many current initiatives favor dividing the risk pool into independent managed-care plans and instituting medical savings accounts based on fixed contributions from government, with high deductibles for beneficiaries. This approach would limit the cost to government and place a higher cost burden on patients. Such plans are being advanced as a positive development because they would make Medicare more like commercial insurance. Ironically, they come at a time when commercial insurance is reducing coverage, raising premiums, and shifting costs to patients. Following the commercial market would actually reduce the sense of security. The introduction of such market-based proposals raises the question of whether we are losing the solidarity that underlies Medicare's success.

When policy analysts from other countries are asked to name the most important feature supporting their universal health-care systems, they typically name social solidarity. The collective will to make the system work appears to be the most important feature of all. The purpose of social insurance is to redistribute resources to those unable to afford private insurance or rely on personal savings, while protecting everyone according to need. Medicare follows this plan but operates partly through a payroll tax paid by younger people in the workforce to benefit older, retired people. The population is thus split into two groups—one that pays and another that benefits. The will to maintain a social contract for Medicare must recognize the advantages of a universal risk pool, covering a large population under one nationwide plan and ultimately benefiting everyone, while also accepting that the pool involves a transfer of resources across generations. There are problems in both of these areas that deserve closer attention.

RISK SOLIDARITY

Pooling health risks has always been a problem in the private market for health insurance. Even community-rated group policies target only a segment of the population, favoring workers, who are evidently at least healthy enough to make it to work. The growth of experience rating in health insurance over the last fifty years has added pressure to segment the risk pool, as indicated by the collapse of the venerable community-rated Blues plans. Individually, healthy people want to pay less, and they typically cost less to insure. Once a serious illness occurs, however, an individual is stigmatized with a preexisting condition and faces skyrocketing premiums. This difficulty in providing affordable insurance for people with severe and chronic conditions is a primary reason for developing a social contract for health.

Transferring resources from the healthy to the unhealthy looks like a standard feature of health insurance, but the practice of underwriting—the basis of experience rating—classifies people into separate risk categories, moderating the transfer. Under experience rating, risk is directly related to price, and resources are shifted from the lucky to the unlucky within the group.[22] This is different from risk solidarity, which balances costs between those with low and high risks.

Charging higher premiums for higher risks looks appropriate with, for instance, automobile insurance, because unsafe driving is demonstrably responsible for higher costs. The same kind of segmentation of risks and premiums looks less appropriate for health care for the following reasons:

1. Most illnesses are not within a person's control;

2. Costs are much greater for health insurance and cannot be avoided, as one might avoid auto insurance costs by simply choosing not to drive;

3. Prevention and screening are potentially beneficial to everyone, and unaffordable premiums for high risks under experience rating are a barrier to access that is harmful to health and unnecessarily expensive.

If we segment people into risk categories based on health, we make insurance unaffordable for the people who need it most. Risk solidarity requires a mandatory system, however, because, as we have seen, younger and healthier people are otherwise inclined to drop their coverage. Medicare maintains a sustainable insurance pool with risk solidarity by requiring everyone to contribute more or less equally to the program's finances and share benefits more or less equally according to need.

As we have already seen, nearly one-half of all expenditures are spent on only 5 percent of Medicare beneficiaries. Nearly all of the expenditures go to only half of the beneficiaries. The remaining half use only 2 percent of all health care expenditures. The extremely skewed distribution of spending brings home the critical importance of risk solidarity in the social contract. No public program of health insurance can survive on reasonable terms if it is made responsible only for the small proportion of the population that incurs most of the costs. Costs must be distributed evenly across the entire population.

Most companies taking part in Medicare+Choice avoid enrolling or succeed in disenrolling older and sicker patients. Since Medicare's monthly payments to Medicare+Choice plans represent the average costs in an area, a company can make a profit by avoiding patients with complex, expensive needs. The pressure for favorable risk selection is especially intense in investor-owned and publicly traded companies with shareholders who expect profits. Here again we see the irony that managed care allows the flexibility to provide good geriatric medical care, yet the pressures for profit may deny it to those who need it the most.

The age distribution of medical spending was fairly even until the 1970s, when expenditures for the elderly and near elderly began to rise dramatically.[23] By 1987, health-care spending for those aged 65 to 74 was three times that for those aged 35 to 44. For the oldest old, over 85, spending was five times greater. Expenditures are concentrated on those with disabilities and in the last year of life. The higher payment rate for the oldest old, according to other studies, is due entirely to increased spending for skilled-nursing facility and home health services; aggressive treatments are reduced.[24] This point highlights the importance of chronic-care management. Medicare, with its coverage gaps, is failing to fully address this responsibility.

Medicare expansion to those under age sixty-five with disabilities and end-stage renal disease (ESRD) confuses the issue of risk solidarity. Average annual spending per disabled nonelderly beneficiary is a bit less than the average for elderly beneficiaries, calculated at $4,663 in 1998; but for beneficiaries with ESRD, two-thirds of whom are under sixty-five, average spending was $30,372.[25] Managing this expense is difficult when co-morbidities and causal health factors in kidney disease, like diabetes and hypertension, remain outside the purview of the program. If younger people had health insurance to cover their diabetes care, fewer would suffer kidney disease requiring Medicare ESRD coverage. Here, Medicare fails in risk solidarity by accepting catastrophic cases without incorporating medical management for the entire nonelderly population.

GENERATIONAL SOLIDARITY

At any point in time, Medicare is clearly transferring funds directly from the young to the old, but the social contract is more complex than this snapshot view suggests. For one thing, a generation is an abstraction. We live in families, not generations. Medicare redistributes resources within families, lightening their overall financial burden considerably. Social insurance for the elderly allows families to redirect private resources to their children. For another, the social contract is an expectation for the future. The fairness of Medicare rests on two important points: first, every working person should expect to receive Medicare benefits on reaching age sixty-five, meaning that the tax payment is like an investment with attached rights, rather than a charitable contribution; and second, working people are spared the burden of paying for much of the health care for their older relatives, and their own security is enhanced by the increased security of their older family members. The concept of generation acquires a definite meaning in an individual's own life. Like Social Security, Medicare is a medical pension that transfers resources from one phase of life to another. The continuity this implies depends on the trust of today's working people that they can count on Medicare benefits for themselves. Retaining this trust is a serious challenge for today's political leaders.

The life-cycle perspective contrasts with references to altruism as the basis of the Medicare program. Altruism is not a social contract. A contract is shaped by a commitment and an explicit recognition of mutual benefits. Although charity is an important human value, the need for it signals a deficiency in the social contract. As society advances, contracts and covenants replace charity as a means to promote justice, allowing altruism to direct its energies to goals beyond supplying the bare necessities of existence.

Seen in this way, the so-called transfer from young to old is not a transfer at all, since current contributions correspond to an expectation of future benefits. For generational solidarity, the relationship is not between young and old in the present, but between young workers today and young workers in the future, as well as their older selves in that same future. The stability of this relationship allows continuity in our social framework. In this case, since future generations have no say in the matter, solidarity means avoiding an unfair transfer of liabilities into the future.

The burden of future insurance liabilities is commonly misjudged and underappreciated in the private market. Insolvencies and retraction of benefits are a frequent result. Social insurance is on firmer ground because of government power to tax to restore reserves, but it also bears a greater risk, because insolvency is not an option and retracting benefits is unjust. Even Medicare needs to conform to sound insurance principles. The prospect of exploding costs has generated enormous efforts at cost control; increasing taxes is a less palatable alternative. However, the political rhetoric assailing taxes tends to ignore the extraordinary benefits that have been gained from Medicare. Of course we need better quality controls, better coordination, and ways to limit unnecessary expenditures; but the expectations of health, maintenance of function, and reduced fear of suffering at the end of life are worth a great deal to the vast majority of the nation's families.

Very little attention is being given to the simple fact that current contributions through the payroll system are inadequate for covering promised benefits in the future. The remedy is simple. The very modest tax that funds Medicare needs to be raised immediately to a reasonable level. A study of generational accounting demonstrates that the unfunded liabilities in Medicare will transfer heavier burdens to future generations and quickly become impossible to sustain.[26] On a positive note, Medicare exhibits less imbalance than similar schemes in many other countries. The same study shows that, among a selection of leading countries, only Canada appears to have fully funded its generational liabilities.

Another criticism of the generational burdens of Medicare concerns those who become terminally ill before reaching age sixty-five, and after paying into the fund find they have no right to health care when they really need it. This anomalous situation is contrary to the inclusivity of social insurance, in which payment creates a right to benefits. Part of the problem here is that Medicare itself is an anomaly, a fallback position from the original goal for universal health insurance.[27]

Finally, respect for generational solidarity highlights the importance of health promotion throughout life. Health promotion will relieve future cost pressures and prevent abuse of the trust of future generations paying the bills. While this goal may be beyond the scope of Medicare, it represents a kind of transfer that deserves responsible management under the social contract. Reducing functional decline and disability should be a major health policy goal of the twenty-first century.

A New Contract for Medicare

Citizens of the United States are often characterized as people who value self-reliance, independence, and free enterprise. Yet our ability to enjoy certain liberties, independence, and economic freedoms depends on the stability provided by a civil society. This becomes abundantly clear as we see democracies around the world foundering when civil society disintegrates. We need government not only to create an environment of respect for the law but also to produce and maintain the infrastructure that allows freedom, productivity, responsibility, and quality of life.

Medicare originated under a principle of income security, offering a measure of relief under a social contract that is increasingly criticized for its failures. The mission of Medicare needs urgently to expand to develop a social contract for health security. Achieving this goal will strengthen society and bring generations together by better supporting families. Health is an essential component of independence and quality of life for all of us, especially as we grow older. We must be able to trust that the system will meet our needs.

The expense of health care makes it impossible for most people to bear the costs of catastrophic illness. Medicare makes a necessary and valuable addition to our civil society by reducing risk and suffering. If we can fix the problems with Medicare and accept that good geriatric and preventive care is an economy rather than an extravagance, Medicare will serve as the model for expanding coverage to younger age groups. What we need to prove, however, is that we have the will and the capacity to proceed further, providing health security not only for the elderly and disabled but for all citizens. By building on its continuing success and enduring popularity, Medicare can serve as a model for developing a new social contract for health that includes everyone.

Glossary

Capitation	A flat, per-month payment to a health-care provider based on the number of individuals served. The fee, which is paid in advance, pays for all of the health-care services provided to insured patients. Capitation allows flexibility in services provided.
Care management	Management of care that addresses multiple needs, including both medical and functional problems. Care management is better suited to management of geriatric conditions than is disease management.
CMS	Centers for Medicare and Medicaid Services. A federal agency within the U.S. Department of Health and Human Services. Before 2001, the agency was known as the Health Care Financing Administration (HCFA).
Disease management	A systematic approach to managing the care of single chronic diseases, usually involving improved care coordination and patient education.
DRG	Diagnosis-related group. A classification system that groups patients by diagnosis, type of treatment, age, or other criteria. Under a prospective payment system (PPS), hospitals are paid based on DRG rather than on hospital charges.
Evidence-based medicine	An approach in which medical decisions about diagnosis and treatment are based on systematically

examined scientific evidence, derived from synthesizing all research studies in a certain area. Many medical interventions have not been tested in this way.

FDA   Food and Drug Administration. A division of the United States Department of Health and Human Services that regulates the safety of drugs, food, medical devices, and other products.

FFS   Fee-for-service. A payment based on the specific service that has been provided. Only specified services are covered in fee-for-service plans.

HMO   Health maintenance organization. A system that provides medical treatment financed by capitation, i.e. on a prepaid basis for a fixed monthly fee, regardless of how many services are actually delivered during the month.

Hospice   A health-care service program based on a philosophy of care that recognizes death as the final stage of life and focuses on improving the quality of life through pain management, family involvement, and holistic care.

Managed care   A range of health plans that impose limits on services covered and use capitation and other economic incentives to hold down costs. The term sometimes refers to integrated delivery systems and sometimes to insurance company approaches to limiting coverage. Managed care can be a method of reducing the costs of unnecessary (not evidence-based) care.

MCO   Managed care organization. A system that combines health-care delivery and financing.

Medicare   The federal payment system for health care that includes:

Part A   Coverage for inpatient hospital expenses, skilled nursing care, some home-health agency services, and hospice care.

Part B   Coverage for outpatient hospital expenses, physician fees, and durable medical equipment.

Part D   Coverage for prescription drugs.

Medicare + Choice	Prepaid health coverage in which Medicare pays monthly fees to HMOs that agree to cover a defined set of services, including Parts A and B. Now called Medicare Advantage.
MediGap	Health insurance sold by private insurance companies to fill "gaps" in Medicare coverage.
PACE	Program of All-Inclusive Care for the Elderly. A program that combines medical, social, and long-term care services for frail people, with the goal of maintaining their independence in their own community. This is the only program in which Medicare (combined with Medicaid) can cover long-term care.
PhRMA	Pharmaceutical Research and Manufacturers of America. A national trade organization for the pharmaceutical industry.
PPO	Preferred-provider organization. A broad network of health-care providers (physicians or physicians and hospitals), linked together for payment of services. Such networks usually do not have integrated medical records or care management.
PPS	Prospective payment system. A system of Medicare reimbursement for Part A benefits that bases most hospital payments on the patient's diagnosis at the time of hospital admission.
PSO	Provider-sponsored organization. A system of providers who are capable of bearing risk *and* delivering a full range of services. No insurance carrier or other intermediary is involved.
RUG	Resource utilization group. A system that sets payment based on the resources expected to be used to care for a nursing home resident, similar to DRGs for hospitals.
SNF	Skilled nursing facility. A facility with staff and equipment to provide skilled nursing care and/or rehabilitation services.

Notes

Introduction

1. The Commonwealth Fund, *2005 Chartbook on Medicare*, www.cmwf.org; Sheila Leatherman and Douglas McCarthy, *Quality of Health Care for Medicare Beneficiaries: A Chartbook* (New York: Commonwealth Fund, 2005).

2. Institute of Medicine, *To Err Is Human: Building a Safer Health System* (Washington, DC: National Academies Press, 1999); Institute of Medicine, *Crossing the Quality Chasm: A New Health System for the 21st Century* (Washington, DC: National Academies Press, 2001).

Chapter 1. Medicare and the Social Contract

1. David Lawrence, *Chaos to Care* (Cambridge, MA: Perseus, 2002), 84.

2. Alliance for Aging Research, *Will You Still Treat Me When I'm 65? The National Shortage of Geriatricians*, 1996, www.agingresearch.org/brochures/treatme /treatme.html, accessed August 3, 2003.

3. Eugene Feingold, *Medicare: Policy and Politics* (San Francisco: Chandler, 1966), 78; House Special Committee on Aging, *Background Facts on the Financing of the Health Care of the Aged*, 87th Cong., 2nd sess., 1962.

4. Theodore Marmor, *The Politics of Medicare*, 2nd ed. (New York: Aldine de Gruyter, 2000), 13.

5. Marmor, *Politics of Medicare*; Jonathan Oberlander, *The Political Life of Medicare* (Chicago: University of Chicago Press, 2003).

6. Quoted in Rosemary Stevens and Robert D. Reischauer, *Medicare and the American Social Contract, Final Report of the Study Panel on Medicare's Larger Social Role* (Washington, DC.: National Academy of Social Insurance, 1999), 3.

7. Stevens and Reischauer, *Medicare and the American Social Contract*.

8. Social Security and Medicare Boards of Trustees, *Status of the Social Security and Medicare Programs: A Summary of the 2004 Annual Reports*, www.ssa.gov/OACT/TRSUM/trsummary.html, accessed April 4, 2005.

9. Ibid.

10. The Physicians' Working Group for Single-Payer National Health Insurance, "Proposal of the Physicians' Working Group for Single-Payer National Health Insurance," *Journal of the American Medical Association* 260, no. 6 (2003): 798–805.

Chapter 2. Longevity and Health

1. John Rowe and Robert L. Kahn, *Successful Aging* (New York: Pantheon, 1998).

2. Frank B. Hobbs and Bonnie L. Damon, *65+ in the United States* (Washington, DC: Bureau of the Census, National Institute on Aging, 1996).

3. U.S. Bureau of the Census, *Middle-Series Projections*, www.census.gov/population/www/projections/popproj.html, accessed April 23, 2003.

4. Constance A. Krach and Victoria A. Velkoff, *Centenarians in the United States*, Current Population Reports, Series P23–199RV (Washington, DC: U.S. Bureau of the Census, 1999), www.census.gov/prod/99pubs/p23–199.pdf, accessed August 2, 2003.

5. Thomas T. Perls, *Who Are Centenarians?* Boston University Medical Campus, www.bumc.bu.edu/Departments/PageMain.asp?Page=5749&DepartmentID=361, accessed April 21, 2003.

6. Margaret B. Neal and Leslie B. Hammer, *Working Couples Caring for Children and Aging Parents: Effects on Work and Well-Being* (Mahwah, NJ: Lawrence Erlbaum, forthcoming).

7. John O. Holloszy, "The Biology of Aging," *Mayo Clinic Proceedings* 75 (January 2000 supplement): S3–S8, S8–S9.

8. Robert Ladislas, "Cellular and Molecular Mechanisms of Aging and Age-Related Diseases," *Pathology and Oncology Research* 6, no. 1 (2000): 3–9.

9. Jeffrey O. Hollinger, Shelley Winn, and Jeffrey Bonadio, "Options for Tissue Engineering to Address Challenges of the Aging Skeleton," *Tissue Engineering* 6, no. 4 (2000): 341–50.

10. Sherine Gabriel, "Update on Epidemiology of the Rheumatic Diseases," *Current Opinion in Rheumatology* 8, no. 2 (1996): 97.

11. Bruce G. Evans and Eduardo D. Salvati, "Total Hip Replacement in the Elderly: Cost-Effective Alternatives," *Instructional Course Lectures* 43 (1994): 359–65.

12. Marc R. Blackman et al., "Growth Hormone and Sex Steroid Administration in Healthy Aged Women and Men: A Randomized Controlled Trial," *Journal of the American Medical Association* 288, no. 18 (2002): 2282–92.

13. Edward D. Zanders, "Impact of Genomics on Medicine," *Pharmacogenomics* 3, no. 4 (2002): 443–46.

14. Steve Salvatore, "Many Triumphs Predicted in War on Cancer: Explosion of New Therapies in Drug Pipeline," CNN, www.cnn.com/2000/HEALTH/Cancer/01/03/cancer, accessed August 2, 2003.

15. Leslie Roberts, "The Gene Hunters: Unlocking the Secrets of DNA to Cure Disease, Slow Aging," *U.S. News and World Report,* January 3, 2000, 34.

16. Eduardo A. Santiago-Delphin, "Transplantation in the Elderly: Changing Philosophy," *Transplantation Proceedings* 28, no. 6 (1996): 3408.

17. Byers W. Shaw, "Transplantation in the Elderly Patient," *Surgical Clinics of North America* 74, no. 2 (1994): 389–400.

18. Mark F. O'Brien et al., "The Medtronic Intact Xenograft: An Analysis of 342 Patients over a Seven-Year Follow-up Period," *Annals of Thoracic Surgery* 60, 2 suppl. (1995) S253–57.

19. Byron Hoogwerf, Atul C. Mehta, and Sethu K. Reddy, "Advances in the Treatment of Diabetes Mellitus in the Elderly: Development of Insulin Analogues," *Drugs and Aging* 9, no. 6 (1996): 438–48.

20. Ernst Chantelau et al., "Effect of Patient-Selected Intensive Insulin Therapy on Quality of Life," *Patient Education and Counseling* 30, no. 2 (1997): 167–73.

21. Kevin Docherty, "Gene Therapy for Diabetes Mellitus," *Clinical Science* 92, no. 4 (1997): 321–30.

22. Graydon S. Meneilly and Daniel Tessier, "Diabetes in the Elderly," *Diabetic Medicine* 12, no. 11 (1995): 949.

23. Nirupama Talwalkar et al., "Outcome of Isolated Coronary Artery Bypass Surgery in Octogenarians," *Journal of Cardiac Surgery* 11, no. 3 (1996): 172–79.

24. Bruce P. Rosenthal, "Changes and Diseases of the Aging Eye," in *Geriatric Medicine,* 4th ed., ed. Christine K. Cassel et al. (New York: Springer, 2003).

25. Kang Zhang et al., "Genetic and Molecular Studies of Macular Dystrophies: Recent Developments," *Survey of Ophthalmology* 40, no. 1 (1995), 51–61.

26. Andrea B. Bodnar et al., "Extension of Life-Span by Introduction of Telomerase into Normal Human Cells," *Science* 279, no. 5349 (January 1998): 349–52.

27. David C. Kelsall, Jon K. Shallop, and Teresa Burnelli, "Cochlear Implantation in the Elderly," *American Journal of Otology* 16, no. 5 (1995): 609–15.

28. Angela Coulter and Chris Ham, *The Global Challenge of Health Care Rationing* (Philadelphia: Open University Press, 2000).

Chapter 3. Ensuring Quality of Care

1. Institute of Medicine, *Crossing the Quality Chasm: A New Health System for the 21st Century* (Washington, DC: National Academies Press, 2001).

2. Paul Starr, "Smart Technology, Stunted Policy: Developing Health Information Networks," *Health Affairs* 16, no. 3 (1997): 91–105.

3. First Consulting Group, *A Primer on Physician Order Entry,* California Healthcare Foundation, 2000, www.fcg.com/webfiles/pdfs/CPOE_Report.pdf, accessed May 8, 2003.

4. National Committee on Vital and Health Statistics, *Information for Health: A Strategy for Building the National Health Information Infrastructure* (Washington, DC: U.S. Department of Health and Human Services, 2001), www.ncvhs.hhs.gov/reptrecs.htm, accessed May 8, 2003.

5. John W. Bachman, "The Patient-Computer Interview: A Neglected Tool That Can Aid the Clinician," *Mayo Clinic Proceedings* 78 (2003): 67–78.

6. Institute of Medicine, *Leadership by Example: Coordinating Government Roles in Improving Health Care Quality* (Washington, DC: National Academies Press, 2002).

7. Kaiser-Permanente Northwest Division, "The Comprehensive Computer-Based Patient Record (CPR)," *Permanente Journal* 3, no. 2 (1999): 13–24.

8. Jeff Goldsmith, "Integrating Care: A Talk with Kaiser Permanente's David Lawrence," *Health Affairs* 21, no. 1 (2002): 39–48.

9. Jack Jue and Anthony F. Jerant, "Six Easy Steps to a Low-Cost Electronic Medical Record," *Family Practice Management,* May 2001, 33–38; M. Lee Chambliss et al., "The Mini Electronic Medical Record: A Low-Cost, Low-Risk Partial Solution," *Journal of Family Practice* 50, no. 12 (2001): 1063–65.

10. Cara B. Litvin et al., "Quality Improvement Using Electronic Medical Records: A Case Study of a High-Performing Practice," *Topics in Health Information Management* 22, no. 2 (2001): 59–64.

11. According to Carolyn Clancy, director of the Agency for Healthcare Research and Quality, and Thomas Scully, administrator of CMS, the Department of Health and Human Services "is poised to promote the adoption of IT standards." See Carolyn M. Clancy and Thomas Scully, "A Call to Excellence," *Health Affairs* 22, no. 2 (2003): 114.

12. Institute of Medicine, *Priority Areas for National Action: Transforming Health Care Quality* (Washington, DC: National Academies Press, 2003).

13. Jennifer L. Wolff, Barbara Starfield, and Gerard Anderson, "Prevalence, Expenditures, and Complications of Multiple Chronic Conditions in the Elderly," *Archives of Internal Medicine* 162 (November 11, 2002): 2269–76.

14. This phrase is drawn from Ralph W. Muller, a participant at the 2002 Duke Health Sector Conference, in *Enabling Prospective Health Care,* ed. Ralph Snyderman and Vicki Y. Saito (Durham, NC: Duke University Medical Center and Health System, 2002), 58.

15. 1999 Physician Masterfile of the American Medical Association. This document is widely available, but it must be purchased from the AMA.

16. Cf. Edward H. Wagner et al., "Improving Chronic Illness Care: Translating Evidence into Action," *Health Affairs* 20, no. 6 (2001): 64–78.

17. See, for example, James W. Kinn et al., "Effectiveness of the Electronic Medical Record in Cholesterol Management in Patients with Coronary Artery Disease (Virtual Lipid Clinic)," *American Journal of Cardiology* 88, no. 2 (2001): 163–65.

18. Hagop S. Mekhjian, "Immediate Benefits Realized following Implementation of Physician Order Entry at an Academic Medical Center," *Journal of the American Medical Informatics Association* 9, no. 5 (2002): 529–39.

19. Sarah Burch, "Evaluating Health Interventions for Older People," *Health* 3, no. 2 (1999): 151–66; David C. Hadorn, "Kinds of Patients," *Journal of Medicine and Philosophy* 22 (1997): 567–87.

20. Stephen E. Ross and Chen-Tan Lin, "The Effects of Promoting Patient Access to Medical Records: A Review," *Journal of the American Medical Informatics Association* 10, no. 2 (2003): 129–38.

21. National Committee on Vital and Health Statistics, *Information for Health*.

22. Elizabeth Goldstein, "CMS's Consumer Information Efforts," *Health Care Financing Review* 23, no. 1 (2001): 1–4.

23. Thomas Scully, "The Changing World of Health Care," in Snyderman and Saito, *Enabling Prospective Health Care*, 109.

24. Institute of Medicine, *Priority Areas for National Action*.

25. Robert Jantzen and Patricia R. Loubeau, "Hospital Selection by Managed Care Insurers," *Health Care Management Review* 25, no. 2 (2000): 93–102.

26. Judith H. Hibbard, Jean Stockard, and Martin Tusler, "Does Publicizing Hospital Performance Stimulate Quality Improvement Efforts?" *Health Affairs* 22, no. 2 (2003): 84–94.

27. Ateev Mehrotra, Thomas Bodenheimer, and Adam Dudley, "Employers' Efforts to Measure and Improve Hospital Quality: Determinants of Success," *Health Affairs* 22, no. 2 (2002): 60–71; David Dranove et al., *Is More Information Better? The Effects of "Report Cards" on Health Care Providers*, working paper 8697 (Cambridge, MA: National Bureau of Economic Research, 2002).

28. William M. Sage, *Accountability through Information: What the Health Care Industry Can Learn from Securities Regulation* (New York: Milbank Memorial Fund, 2000); Donald M. Berwick, Brent James, and Molly Joel Coye, "Connections between Quality Measurement and Improvement," *Medical Care* 41, supplement 1 (2003): I30–I38.

29. E. S. Fisher, D. E. Wennberg, T. A. Stukel, M. S. Gottlieb, F. L. Lucas, and E. L. Pinder, "The Implications of Regional Variations in Medicare Spending, Part 1: The Content, Quality, and Accessibility of Care," *Annals of Internal Medicine* 138 (2003): 273–87.

30. Ibid.

31. K. I. Shine, "Geographical Variations in Medicare Spending," *Annals of Internal Medicine* 138 (2003): 347.

32. For an elaboration of these principles, see Christine K. Cassel, Rosanne Leipzig, Harvey Jay Cohen, Eric B. Larson, and Diane E. Meier, eds., *Geriatric Medicine,* 4th ed. (New York: Springer, 2003).

Chapter 4. Care Management

1. See Mark S. Lachs and Hirsch S. Ruchlin, "Is Managed Care Good or Bad for Geriatric Medicine?" *Journal of the American Geriatrics Society* 45, no. 9 (1997): 1123–27.

2. Alliance for Aging Research, *Will You Still Treat Me When I'm 65? The Na-*

tional Shortage of Geriatricians, 1996, www.agingresearch.org/brochures/treatme/treatme.html, accessed August 3, 2003.

3. Institute of Medicine, "Appendix C: Technical Overview: Health System Information Systems of VHA and DOD," in *Leadership by Example* (Washington, DC: National Academies Press, 2002).

4. Brian Biles, Geraldine Dallek, and Andrew Dennington, *Medicare+Choice after Five Years: Lessons for Medicare's Future* (New York: Commonwealth Fund, 2002).

5. Richard Kronick and Joy de Beyer, "The Problem of Selection in Medicare Risk-Contract HMOs," in *Medicare HMOs: Making Them Work for the Chronically Ill,* ed. Richard Kronick and Joy de Beyer (Chicago: Health Administration Press, 1999), 9–26.

6. Roberto Bernabei et al., "Randomized Trial of Impact of Model of Integrated Care and Case Management for Older People Living in the Community," *British Medical Journal* 316 (May 2, 1998):1348–51; Francesco Landi et al., "Impact of Integrated Home Care Services on Hospital Use," *Journal of the American Geriatrics Society* 47, no. 12 (1999): 1430–34; Brenda S. Marshall et al., "Case Management of the Elderly in a Health Maintenance Organization: The Implications for Program Administration under Managed Care," *Journal of Healthcare Management* 44, no. 6 (1999): 477–491; Anita J. Gagnon et al., "Randomized Controlled Trial of Nurse Case Management of Frail Older People," *Journal of the American Geriatrics Society* 47, no. 9 (1999): 1118–24; Chad Boult et al., "Does Case Management Save Money in Medicare HMOs?" paper presented at the Annual Scientific Meeting of the American Geriatrics Society and American Federation for Aging Research, Nashville, TN, May 2000.

7. Barbara Starfield and Thomas Oliver, "Primary Care in the United States and Its Precarious Future," *Health and Social Care in the Community* 7, no. 5 (1999): 315–23.

8. Peter D. Fox, "Applying Managed Care to Medicare," *Health Affairs* 16, no. 5 (1997), 44–57.

9. Lisa Yount, *Patients' Rights in the Age of Managed Care* (New York: Facts on File, 2001); Muriel R. Gillick, "Medicare Coverage for Technological Innovations—Time for New Criteria?" *New England Journal of Medicine* 350, no. 21 (2004), 2199–2203.

10. Edward H. Wagner, "Care of Older People with Chronic Illness," in *New Ways to Care for Older People: Building Systems Based on Evidence,* ed. Evan Calkins et al. (New York: Springer, 1999).

11. Pam Silberman et al., "Tracking Medicaid Managed Care in Rural Communities: A Fifty-State Follow-up," *Health Affairs* 21, no. 4 (2002): 255–263.

12. Mathematica Policy Research, *Best Practices in Coordinated Care,* contract no. HCFA 500–95–0048 (04), (Baltimore, MD: Health Care Financing Administration, Division of Demonstration Programs, 2000).

13. Ibid., 2.

14. Kenneth G. Manton and XiLiang Gu, "Changes in the Prevalence of Chronic Disability in the United States Black and Nonblack Population above

Age 65 from 1982 to 1999," *Proceedings of the National Academy of Sciences* 98, no. 11 (2001): 6354–59.

15. Judith Feder and Jeanne Lambrew, "Why Medicare Matters to People Who Need Long-Term Care," *Health Care Financing Review* 18, no. 2 (1996): 99–112.

16. See David Blumenthal et al., eds., *Long-Term Care and Medicare Policy: Can We Improve the Continuity of Care?* (Washington, DC: National Academy of Social Insurance, 2003).

17. Centers for Medicare and Medicaid Services, *Program of All Inclusive Care for the Elderly,* www.medicare.gov/Nursing/Alternatives/Pace.asp, accessed August 2, 2003.

18. Catherine Eng et al., "Program of All-Inclusive Care for the Elderly (PACE): An Innovative Model of Integrated Geriatric Care and Financing," *Journal of the American Geriatrics Society* 45, no. 2 (1997): 223–32.

19. MedPAC, "Managed Care for Frail Medicare Beneficiaries: Payment Methods and Program Standards," in *Report to Congress: Medicare Payment Policy* (Washington, DC, 1999); Abt Associates, *Evaluation of the Program of All-Inclusive Care for the Elderly (PACE) Demonstration: The Impact of PACE on Participant Outcomes,* HCFA contract no. 500–96–0003/T04 (Baltimore MD: Health Care Financing Administration, Office of Strategic Planning, 1998).

Chapter 5. Palliative Care

1. John W. Rowe and Robert L. Kahn, *Successful Aging* (New York: Pantheon, 1998).

2. National Center for Health Statistics, *Deaths by Place of Death, Age, Race, and Sex: United States, 1999–2001,* www.cdc.gov/nchs/datawh/statab/unpubd/mortabs/gmwk309_10.htm, accessed April 24, 2003; Joanne Lynne, *Sick to Death and Not Going to Take It Anymore! Reforming Health Care for the Last Years of Life* (Berkeley: University of California Press, 2004).

3. National Hospice and Palliative Care Organization, *NHPCO Facts and Figures,* www.nhpco.org, accessed April 24, 2003.

4. MedPAC, *Report to the Congress: Medicare Beneficiaries' Access to Hospice* (Washington, DC.: Medicare Payment Advisory Commission, 2002).

5. James S. Larson and Krista K. Larson, "Evaluating End-of-Life Care from the Perspective of the Patient's Family," *Evaluation and the Health Professions* 25, no. 2 (2002): 143–51.

6. Carol P. Curtiss, "JCAHO: Meeting the Standards for Pain Management," *Orthopaedic Nursing* 20, no. 2 (2001): 27–30, 41.

7. Last Acts, *Means to a Better End: A Report on Dying in America Today* (Washington, DC: Last Acts National Program Office, 2002).

8. Center to Advance Palliative Care, "Palliative Care Programs Rapidly Growing in Nation's Hospitals," press release, January 2, 2003, www.capc.org/content/278, accessed April 24, 2003.

9. Cynthia X. Pan et al., " How Prevalent Are Hospital-Based Palliative Care

Programs? Status Report and Future Directions," *Journal of Palliative Medicine* 4, no. 3 (2001): 315–24.

10. The SUPPORT Principal Investigators, "A Controlled Trial to Improve Care for Seriously Ill Hospitalized Patients: The Study to Understand Prognoses and Preferences for Outcomes and Risks of Treatments (SUPPORT)," *JAMA*, 274 (1995): 1591–98.

11. Dartmouth Medical School, Center for Evaluative Study, *The Dartmouth Atlas of Health Care 1999*, ed. John E. Wennberg (Washington, DC: AHA Press, 1999).

12. Timothy J. Keay, "Palliative Care in the Nursing Home," *Generations* 23, no. 1 (1999): 96–98.

13. Jerome Groopman, *Second Opinions* (New York: Viking, 2000); Jerome Groopman, *The Measure of Our Days: New Beginnings at Life's End* (New York: Viking, 1997).

14. Roberto Barnabei et al., "Management of Pain in Elderly Patients with Cancer," *Journal of the American Medical Association* 279, no. 23 (1998): 1877–82.

15. AGS Panel on Chronic Pain in Older Persons, "The Management of Chronic Pain in Older Persons," *Journal of the American Geriatrics Society* 46, no. 5 (1998): 635–51.

16. Karen S. Feldt, Muriel B. Ryden, and Steven Miles, "Treatment of Pain in Cognitively Impaired Compared with Cognitively Intact Older Patients with Hip Fracture," *Journal of the American Geriatrics Society* 46, no. 9 (1998): 1079–85.

17. Institute of Medicine, *Approaching Death: Improving Care at the End of Life*, ed. Marilyn J. Field and Christine K. Cassel (Washington, DC: National Academies Press, 1997).

Chapter 6. Medicare Coverage

1. Lawrence R. Jacobs, *The Health of Nations: Public Opinion and The Making of American and British Health Policy* (Ithaca, NY: Cornell University Press, 1993), 87.

2. Theodore Marmor, *The Politics of Medicare,* 2nd ed. (New York: Aldine de Gruyter, 2000), 12.

3. Jacobs, *The Health of Nations,* 100.

4. Medicare coverage rules are scrupulously posted and easily accessed on the CMS website (www.medicare.gov).

5. Robert M. Ball, "Social Insurance Commentary," in *Medicare: Preparing for the Challenge of the 21st Century,* ed. Robert D. Reischauer, Stuart Butler, and Judith Lave (Washington, DC: Brookings Institution Press, 1998), 27–37.

6. Marilyn Moon, *Medicare Now and in the Future,* 2nd ed. (Washington, DC: Urban Institute Press, 1996).

7. Oregon Health Policy and Research, *Oregon HRSA State Planning Grant: Final Report to the Secretary,* 2001, http://www.ohpr.org/hrsa/Finalreport/Sect3-10-27.pdf, accessed April 28, 2003.

8. Health Care Financing Administration, "Medicare Program: Procedures for Making National Coverage Decisions," HCFA, 3432-GN, *Federal Register* 64, no. 80 (April 27, 1999): 22619–25 [FR Doc. 99–10460].

9. Vicki Gottlich, *Medical Necessity Determinations in the Medicare Program: Are the Interests of Beneficiaries with Chronic Conditions Being Met?* (Baltimore, MD: Johns Hopkins University and the Robert Wood Johnson Foundation, 2003).

10. Susan Bartlett Foote, "Why Medicare Cannot Promulgate a National Coverage Rule: A Case of Regula Mortis," *Journal of Health Politics, Policy, and Law* 27, no. 5 (2002): 707–30.

11. Phillip W. Beatty and Kelley R. Dhont, "Medicare Health Maintenance Organizations and Traditional Coverage: Perceptions of Health Care among Beneficiaries with Disabilities," *Archives of Physical Medicine and Rehabilitation* 82, no. 8 (2001): 1009–17.

12. Marilyn Moon, "Medicare Matters: Building on a Record of Accomplishments," *Health Care Financing Review* 22, no. 1 (2000): 9–22.

13. Stephanie Maxwell, Matthew Storeygard, and Marilyn Moon, *Modernizing Medicare Cost-Sharing: Policy Options and Impacts on Beneficiary and Program Expenditures* (New York: Commonwealth Fund, 2002).

14. Kaiser Family Foundation, *Medicare Chart Book,* 2nd ed. (Menlo Park, CA: Kaiser Family Foundation, 2001).

15. Ibid.

16. Nora Super, *Medigap: Prevalence, Premiums, and Opportunities for Reform,* NHPF Issue Brief No. 782 (Washington, DC: National Health Policy Forum, 2002).

17. Kaiser Family Foundation and Hewitt Associates, *The Current State of Retiree Health Benefits: Findings from the Kaiser/Hewitt 2002 Retiree Health Survey,* (Menlo Park, CA: Kaiser Family Foundation, 2002).

18. Marsha Gold and Lori Achman, *Average Out-of-Pocket Health Care Costs for Medicare+Choice Enrollees Increase Substantially in 2002,* Issue Brief (New York: Commonwealth Fund, 2002).

19. Rani Snyder, Thomas Rice, and Michelle Kitchman, *Paying for Choice: The Cost Implications of Health Plan Options for People on Medicare* (Menlo Park, CA: Kaiser Family Foundation, 2003).

20. James C. Robinson, "Physician Organization in California: Crisis and Opportunity," *Health Affairs* 20, no. 4 (2001): 81–96; James C. Robinson and Lawrence P. Casalino, "Reevaluation of Capitation Contracting in New York and California," *Health Affairs* web exclusive, www.healthaffairs.org, May 17, 2001, accessed May 1, 2003.

21. Robert Hurley et al., "A Longitudinal Perspective on Health Plan-Provider Risk Contracting," *Health Affairs* 21, no. 4 (2002): 144–53.

22. E. S. Fisher, D. E. Wemberg, T. A. Stukel, et al., *Annals of Internal Medicine* 138, no. 4 (2003): 273–87.

23. Andrew Kramer et al., "Outcome and Utilization Differences for Older Persons with Stroke in HMO and Fee-for-Service Systems," *Journal of the American Geriatrics Society* 48, no. 7 (2000): 726–34.

24. Dana Gelb Safran et al., "Primary Care Quality in the Medicare Program: Comparing the Performance of Medicare Health Maintenance Organizations and Traditional Fee-for-Service Medicare," *Archives of Internal Medicine* 162, no. 7 (2002): 757–65.

25. Richard Kronick and Joy de Beyer, eds., *Medicare HMOs: Making Them Work for the Chronically Ill* (Chicago: Health Administration Press, 1999).

26. Robert Morgan et al., "The Medicare-HMO Revolving Door: The Healthy Go In and the Sick Go Out," *New England Journal of Medicine* 337, no. 3 (1997): 169–75.

27. Department of Health and Human Services, Office of the Inspector General, *Adequacy of Medicare's Managed Care Payments after the Balanced Budget Act of 1997*, A-14–00–00212 (September 18, 2000).

28. Brian Biles, Geraldine Dallek, and Andrew Dennington, *Medicare + Choice After Five Years: Lessons for Medicare's Future* (New York: Commonwealth Fund, 2002).

29. Timothy Lake and Randall Brown, *Medicare + Choice Withdrawals: Understanding Key Factors* (Menlo Park, CA: Kaiser Family Foundation, 2002); Centers for Medicare and Medicaid Services, *Protecting Medicare Beneficiaries When Their Medicare + Choice Organization Withdraws,* 2002, http://cms.hhs.gov/media/press/release.asp?counter=402, accessed April 4, 2005.

30. Jennifer Stuber et al., *Instability and Inequity in Medicare + Choice: The Impact on Medicare Beneficiaries* (New York: Commonwealth Fund, 2002); Geraldine Dallek and Andrew Dennington, *Physician Withdrawals: A Major Source of Instability in the Medicare + Choice Program* (New York: Commonwealth Fund, 2002); Lori Acherman and Marsha Gold, *Medicare + Choice Plans Continue to Shift More Costs to Enrollees* (New York: Commonwealth Fund, 2003).

31. Beth Demel et al., *Systemic Problems with Medicare HMOs: Case Studies from the Medicare Rights Center HMO Hotline* (New York: Medicare Rights Center), www.medicarerights.org, accessed August 2, 2003.

32. Lori Achman and Marsha Gold, *Medicare + Choice 1999–2001: An Analysis of Managed Care Plan Withdrawals and Trends in Benefits and Premiums* (New York: Commonwealth Fund, 2002).

33. Geraldine Dallek, Andrew Dennington, and Brian Biles, *Geographic Inequity in Medicare + Choice Benefits: Findings from Seven Communities* (New York: Commonwealth Fund, 2002).

34. Hongjun Kan, "Does the Medicare Principal Inpatient Diagnostic Cost Group Model Adequately Adjust for Selection Bias?" Ph.D. diss., Rand Graduate School, 2002, www.rand.org, April 26, 2002.

35. Robert Kuttner, "The Risk-Adjustment Debate," *New England Journal of Medicine* 339, no. 26 (1998): 1952–56.

36. Hongjun Kan, "Does the Medicare Principal Inpatient Diagnostic Cost Group Model Adequately Adjust for Selection Bias?"

37. Mark McClellan and Sontine Kalba, "Benefit Diversity in Medicare: Choice, Competition, and Selection," in Kronick and de Beyer, eds., *Medicare HMOs*, 133–60.

38. Gerard Anderson, "Stronger Oversight and Additional Regulation of Plans," in *Medicare HMOs,* 161–81.

39. Centers for Medicare and Medicaid Services, *Protecting Medicare Beneficiaries.*

40. Alison Evans Cuellar and Joshua M. Wiener, "Can Social Insurance for Long-Term Care Work? The Experience of Germany," *Health Affairs* 19, no. 3 (2000): 8–25.

41. Deborah Stone, "Why Is It So Hard To Do Home Care Right?" paper presented at the Institute for Medicare Practice, Mount Sinai School of Medicine, April 2000.

42. Brett Baker, "Medicare Clarifies Its Definition of 'Homebound,'" *ACP-ASIM Observer,* June 2001, www.acponline.org/journals/news/jun01/q&a.htm, accessed August 2, 2003.

43. Abt Associates, *Evaluation of the Program of All-Inclusive Care for the Elderly Demonstration: Final Report,* Contract No. 500–01–0027 (Washington, DC: Health Care Financing Administration, 2000); Abt Associates, *Evaluation of the Program of All-Inclusive Care for the Elderly (PACE) Demonstration: Final,* Contract No. 500–96–0003/T04 (Washington, DC: Health Care Financing Administration, 1998).

44. CMS OSCAR Data Current Surveys, *Nursing Facility Patients by Payer: Percentage of Patients,* 2002, www.ahca.org/research/oscar/rpt_payer1_dec02.pdf, accessed August 2, 2003.

45. Judith Feder and Jeanne Lambrew, "Why Medicare Matters to People Who Need Long-Term Care," *Health Care Financing Review* 18, no. 2 (1996): 99–112.

46. U.S. General Accounting Office, *Medicare and Medicaid: Implementing State Demonstrations for Dual Eligibles Has Proven Challenging,* GAO/HEHS-00–94 (Washington, DC: United States General Accounting Office, 2000).

47. Ibid.

Chapter 7. Why Sixty-five?

1. Frank R. Lichtenberg, *The Effects of Medicare on Health Care Utilization and Outcomes* (Cambridge, MA: National Bureau of Economic Research, 2001).

2. Hajo Holborn, *A History of Modern Germany, 1840–1945,* vol. 3 (Princeton, NJ: Princeton University Press, 1987).

3. Catherine Hoffman and Alan Schlobohm, *Uninsured in America: A Chartbook,* 2nd ed (Menlo Park, CA: Kaiser Family Foundation, 2000).

4. Institute for Social Research, University of Michigan, 1998, *HRA: Study of Health, Retirement and Aging,* http://hrsonline.isr.umich.edu/news/newsletter/english/news1998e.pdf, accessed July 27, 2003; Institute for Social Research, University of Michigan, *The Health and Retirement Study,* http://hrsonline.isr.umich.edu, accessed April 4, 2005.

5. John Budetti et al., *Risks of Midlife Americans: Getting Sick, Becoming Disabled, or Losing a Job and Health Coverage* (New York: Commonwealth Fund, 2000).

6. Ibid.

7. Robert J. Mills, "Health Insurance Coverage: 2000," *Current Population Reports* (Washington, DC: U.S. Census Bureau, 2001).

8. Hoffman and Schlobohm, *Uninsured in America;* ACP-ASIM, *No Health Insurance? It's Enough to Make You Sick,* 2001, www.acponline.org/uninsured/lack-contents.htm, accessed July 27, 2003; Robert Wood Johnson Foundation, *Annual Report: Americans without Health Insurance: Myths and Realities* (Princeton, NJ: Robert Wood Johnson Foundation, 1999).

9. Hoffman and Schlobohm, *Uninsured in America.*

10. Budetti et al., *Risks of Midlife Americans.*

11. Edward D. Frohlich, "Hypertension," in *Geriatric Medicine*, 2nd ed., ed. Christine K. Cassel et al. (New York: Springer, 1990), 141–51.

12. National Center for Health Statistics, *Health, United States, 1995* (Hyattsville, MD: Public Health Service, 1996).

13. American Heart Association, *Risk Factors and Coronary Heart Disease*, 2000, www.americanheart.org, accessed October 17, 2000.

14. Ali H. Mokdad et al., "Diabetes Trends in the US: 1990–1998," *Diabetes Care* 23, no. 9 (2000): 1278–83.

15. Centers for Disease Control, *Diabetes Public Health Resource: Frequently Asked Questions,* 2000, www.cdc.gov/diabetes/faqs.htm, accessed September 29, 2000.

16. Hoffman and Schlobohm, *Uninsured in America.*

17. National Cancer Institute, *Cancer Facts: Lifetime Probability of Breast Cancer in American Women,* 2002, http://cis.nci.nih.gov/fact/5_6.htm, accessed July 27, 2003.

18. Donald K. Blackman, Eddas M. Bennett, and Daniel S. Miller, "Trends in Self-Reported Use of Mammogram (1989–1997) and Papanicolaou Tests (1991–1997): Behavioral Risk Factor Surveillance System," *MMWR Weekly* 48, no. SS06 (October 8, 1999): 1–22.

19. Ibid.

20. Hoffman and Schlobohm, *Uninsured in America.*

21. Centers for Disease Control, "Osteoporosis among Estrogen-Deficient Women: United States, 1988–1994," *MMWR Weekly* 47, no. 45 (November 20, 1998): 969–73.

22. Institute for Social Research, University of Michigan, *HRA: Study of Health, Retirement and Aging.*

23. National Academy on an Aging Society, *Caregiving: Helping the Elderly with Activity Limitations*, Number 7 (Washington, DC: National Academy on an Aging Society, 2000).

24. Robert C. Morris and Francis G. Caro, "The Young-Old, Productive Aging, and Public Policy," *Generations* 19, no. 3 (1995): 32–37.

25. AARP Public Policy Institute, *Boomers Approaching Midlife: How Secure a Future?* (Washington, DC: AARP, 1998).

26. John W. Rowe and Robert L. Kahn, *Successful Aging* (New York: Pantheon Books, 1998).

Chapter 8. Insurance

1. American Medical Association Center for Health Policy Research, *Physician Socioeconomic Statistics, 1999–2000* (Chicago: American Medical Association, 1999).

2. MedPAC, *Report to the Congress: Medicare Payment Policy* (Washington, DC.: Medicare Payment Advisory Commission, 2003), figures 1–5.

3. Ellen O'Brien and Judith Feder, *Employment-Based Health Insurance Coverage and Its Decline: The Growing Plight of Low-Wage Workers* (Menlo Park, CA: Kaiser Family Foundation, 1999).

4. Kaiser Family Foundation and Health Research and Educational Trust, *Employer Health Benefits: 2002 Annual Survey* (Menlo Park, CA: Kaiser Family Foundation, 2002).

5. Marc L. Berk and Alan C. Monheit, "The Concentration of Health Care Expenditures, Revisited," *Health Affairs* 20, no. 2 (2001): 9–18.

6. Zhou Yang, Edward C. Norton, and Sally C. Stearns, "Longevity and Health Care Expenditures," *Journals of Gerontology, Series B: Psychological Sciences and Social Sciences* 58, no. 1 (2003): S2–S10; Norman G. Levinsky et al., "Influence of Age on Medicare Expenditures and Medical Care in the Last Year of Life," *Journal of the American Medical Association* 286, no. 11 (2001): 1349–55.

7. Frank R. Dobbin, "The Origins of Private Social Insurance: Public Policy and Fringe Benefits in America, 1920–1950," *American Journal of Sociology* 97, no. 5 (1992): 1416–50.

8. Paul Starr, *The Social Transformation of American Medicine* (New York: Basic Books, 1982); James Weinstein, *The Corporate Ideal in the Liberal State, 1900–1918* (Boston: Beacon, 1968).

9. Eugene Feingold, *Medicare: Policy and Politics* (San Francisco: Chandler, 1966).

10. Marilyn Moon, *Medicare Now and In the Future*, 2nd ed. (Washington, DC: Urban Institute, 1996).

11. Mark McClellan, *Medicare and the Federal Budget: Past Experience, Current Policy, Future Prospects* (Cambridge, MA: National Bureau of Economic Research, 2000).

12. Health Care Financing Administration, "Growth in Medicare Program Payments," *Health Care Financing Review* 17, supplement 1 (1995): 38–40.

13. McClellan, *Medicare and the Federal Budget*.

14. Howard Hiatt, "Protecting the Medical Commons: Who Is Responsible?" *New England Journal of Medicine* 293, no. 5 (1975): 235–41.

15. Centers for Medicare and Medicaid Services, *Acute Inpatient Prospective Payment System Related Information*, www.cms.hhs.gov/providers/hipps/default.asp, accessed August 2, 2003.

16. For an analysis suggesting that DRGs did not slow the rate of growth in hospital expenditures, see Ronald J. Vogel, *Medicare: Issues in Political Economy* (Ann Arbor: University of Michigan Press, 1999).

17. Office of the Inspector General, *Medicare Beneficiary Access to Skilled Nursing Facilities* (Washington, DC: U.S. Department of Health and Human Services, 2001).

18. Robert Hurley et al., "A Longitudinal Perspective on Health Plan–Provider Risk Contracting," *Health Affairs* 21, no. 4 (2002): 144–53.

19. Mira Johri, Francois Beland, and Howard Bergman, "International Experiments in Integrated Care for the Elderly: A Synthesis of the Evidence," *International Journal of Geriatric Psychiatry* 18, no. 3 (2003): 222–35.

20. S. A. Schroeder, L. P. Myers, S. J. McPhee, et al., "The Failure of Physician Education as a Cost Containment Strategy," *Journal of the American Medical Association* 252, no. 2 (1984): 225–30.

21. Michael E. Gluck and Kristina W. Hanson, *Medicare Chartbook* (Menlo Park, CA: Kaiser Family Foundation, 2001); Centers for Medicare and Medicaid Services, *Medicare Managed Care Contract Plans Monthly Summary Report* (May 2003), http://cms.hhs.gov/healthplans/statistics/mmcc, accessed May 28, 2003.

22. Liza Greenberg, "Overview: PPO Performance Measurement: Agenda for the Future," *Medical Care Research and Review* 58, supplement 1 (2001): 8–15.

23. Richard Hamer and Deborah Anderson, *PPO Operations and Markets* (Menlo Park, CA: Kaiser Family Foundation, 2000).

24. Alain C. Enthoven, *Theory and Practice of Managed Competition in Health Care Finance* (New York: Elsevier Science, 1988).

25. Thomas R. Oliver, "Analysis, Advice, and Congressional Leadership: The Physician Payment Review Commission and the Politics of Medicare," *Journal of Health Politics, Policy and Law* 18, no. 1 (1993): 113–74.

26. Ibid.

27. Ira Burney and Julia Paradise, "Trends In Medicare Physician Participation and Assignment," *Health Affairs* 6, no. 2 (1987): 107–20.

28. David C. Colby et al., "Balance Billing under Medicare: Protecting Beneficiaries and Preserving Physician Participation," *Journal of Health Politics, Policy, and Law* 20, no. 1 (1995): 49–74.

29. House Committee on Ways and Means, Subcommittee on Health, *Hearing on Medicare Payments to Physicians: Statement of Glenn M. Hackbarth,* 109th Cong., 1st sess., February 10, 2005.

30. Katharine Levit et al., "Trends in U.S. Health Care Spending, 2001," *Health Affairs* 22, no. 1 (2003): 154–64.

31. Health Care Financing Administration, "Medicare Program; Revisions to Payment Policies under the Physician Fee Schedule for Calendar Year 2000, Addendum B: 2000 Relative Value Units and Related Information Used in Determining Medicare Payments for 2000," 42 CFR, parts 410, 411, 414, and 415 [HCFA-1065-P], *Federal Register* 64 (1999): 39642–56.

32. Centers for Medicare and Medicaid Services, "1.2.4. Updating the Work RVUs," in *Five Year Review of Work Relative Value Units (HER),* 2000, www.cms.gov/physicians/pfs/wrvu-ch1.asp, accessed August 2, 2003.

33. AMA Center for Health Policy Research, *Physician Socioeconomic Statistics, 1999–2000,* 10.

34. Sue Cejka, "Physician Compensation in 1998: Both Specialists and Primary Care Physicians Emerge as Winners," *Hospital Physician,* January 2000, 61–68, http://www.turner-white.com/pdf/hp_jan00_phycomp1998.pdf, accessed May 29, 2003.

35. Hsiao et al., "Results and Policy Implications."

36. See L. Elizabeth Sloan, "Fraud, Abuse, and Medicare Billing: Should You Be Worried?" *AACAP News,* July–August 1998, www.aacap.org/clinical/fraud.htm, accessed May 28, 2003.

37. Matthew K. Wynia et al., "Physician Manipulation of Reimbursement Rules for Patients: Between a Rock and a Hard Place," *Journal of the American Medical Association* 283, no. 14 (2000): 1858–65.

38. Cf. J. D. Kleinke, "Deconstructing the Columbia/HCA Investigation," *Health Affairs* 17, no. 2 (1998): 7–26. See also Jeff Goldsmith, Uwe E. Reinhardt, and Bruce C. Vladeck, "Perspectives," in the same issue.

39. Kaiser Family Foundation and Harvard University School of Public Health, *National Survey on Medicare Policy Options,* 1998, www.kff.org/medicare/1442-reform_pr.cfm, accessed April 5, 2005.

Chapter 9. Prescription Drugs

1. Kaiser Family Foundation, *Prescription Drug Trends: A Chartbook Update* (Menlo Park, CA: Kaiser Family Foundation, 2001).

2. S. D. Finlay, "Direct-to-Consumer Promotion of Prescription Drugs: Economic Implications for Patients, Payers and Providers," *PharmacoEconomics* 19, no 2 (2001): 109–19; Kaiser Family Foundation, *Trends and Indicators in the Changing Health Care Marketplace, 2002* (Menlo Park, CA: Kaiser Family Foundation, 2002).

3. J. D. Kleinke, "The Price of Progress: Prescription Drugs in the Health Care Market," *Health Affairs* 20, no. 5 (2001): 43–60.

4. Ernst R. Berndt, "The U.S. Pharmaceutical Industry: Why Major Growth in Times of Cost Containment?" *Health Affairs* 20, no. 2 (2001): 100–114.

5. Kaiser Family Foundation, *Prescription Drug Trends: A Chartbook Update.*

6. John A. Poisal and Lauren Murray, "Growing Differences Between Medicare Beneficiaries With and Without Drug Coverage," *Health Affairs* 20, no. 2 (2001): 74–85.

7. Kaiser Family Foundation and Hewitt Associates, *The Current State of Retiree Health Benefits: Findings from the Kaiser/Hewitt 2002 Retiree Health Survey* (Menlo Park, CA: Kaiser Family Foundation, 2002).

8. Lori Achman and Marsha Gold, *Medicare+Choice 1999–2001: An Analysis of Managed Care Plan Withdrawals and Trends in Benefits and Premiums* (New York: Commonwealth Fund, 2002).

9. Kaiser Family Foundation, *Trends and Indicators.*

10. Kaiser Family Foundation, *Prescription Drug Trends.*

11. Michael S. Wilkes, Robert A. Bell, and Richard L. Kravitz, "Direct-to-Consumer Prescription Drug Advertising: Trends, Impact, and Implications," *Health Affairs* 19, no. 2 (2000): 110–28; Mike Mitka, "Survey Suggesting that Prescription Drug Ads Help Public is Met with Skepticism," *Journal of the American Medical Association* 289, no. 7 (2003): 827–28.

12. Michelle M. Mello, Meredith Rosenthal, and Peter J. Neumann, "Direct-

to-Consumer Advertising and Shared Liability for Pharmaceutical Manufacturers," *Journal of the American Medical Association* 289, no. 4 (2003): 477–81.

13. Robert Pear, "Marketing Tied to Increase In Prescription Drug Sales," *New York Times,* September 20, 2000.

14. Steven Reichert, Todd Simon, and Ethan A. Halm, "Physicians' Attitudes about Prescribing and Knowledge of the Costs of Common Medications," *Archives of Internal Medicine* 160 (October 9, 2000): 2799–803; Michael E. Ernst et al., "Prescription Medication Costs: A Study of Physician Familiarity," *Archives of Family Medicine* 9 (November–December 2000): 1002–7.

15. Lisa M. Korn et al., "Improving Physicians' Knowledge of the Costs of Common Medications and Willingness to Consider Costs When Prescribing," *Journal of General Internal Medicine* 18 (January 2003): 31–37.

16. Michael E. Gluck, *A Medicare Prescription Drug Benefit* (Washington, DC: National Academy of Social Insurance, 1999).

17. Kaiser Family Foundation, *Medicare and Prescription Drugs* (Menlo Park, CA: Kaiser Family Foundation, 2002).

18. See the website of the Medicare Rights Center: www.medicarerights.org.

19. Kaiser Family Foundation, *Seniors and Prescription Drugs* (Menlo Park, CA: Kaiser Family Foundation, 2002).

20. Benjamin M. Craig, David H. Kreling, and David A. Mott, "Do Seniors Get the Medicines Prescribed for Them? Evidence from the 1996–1999 Medicare Current Beneficiary Survey," *Health Affairs* 22, no. 3 (2003): 175–82.

21. Alyce S. Adams, Stephen B. Soumerai, and Dennis Ross-Degnan, "The Case for a Medicare Drug Coverage Benefit: A Critical Review of the Empirical Evidence," *Annual Review of Public Health* 22 (2001): 49–61.

22. Richard G. Frank, "Prescription Drug Prices: Why Do Some Pay More than Others Do?" *Health Affairs* 20, no. 2 (2001): 115–28.

23. Kaiser Family Foundation, *Federal Policies Affecting the Cost and Availability of New Pharmaceuticals* (Menlo Park, CA: Kaiser Family Foundation, 2002).

24. Alan Murray, "Drug Makers' Battle Is One over Ideas," *Wall Street Journal,* March 19, 2001.

25. Jerome Groopman, *Second Opinions* (New York: Viking, 2000).

26. Alain C. Enthoven, *Theory and Practice of Managed Competition in Health Care Finance* (New York: Elsevier Science, 1988).

27. Office for Oregon Health Policy and Research, www.oregonRx.org, accessed November 19, 2004.

28. Daniel M. Fox, "Evidence of Evidence-based Health Policy: The Politics of Systematic Reviews in Coverage Decisions," *Health Affairs* 24, no. 1 (2005): 114–22.

29. David Blumenthal and Roger Herdman, *Description and Analysis of the VA National Formulary* (Washington, DC: National Academies Press, 2000).

30. Panos Kanavos and Uwe Reinhardt, "Reference Pricing for Drugs: Is it Compatible with U.S. Health Care?" *Health Affairs* 22, no. 3 (2003): 16–30.

31. PhRMA, *Do Price Controls Hurt Pharmaceutical Research? Recent History Says "Yes,"* 1999, www.phrma.org/publications, accessed March 19, 2001.

32. Kaiser Family Foundation, *Federal Policies.*

33. Kaiser Family Foundation, *Prescription Drug Trends: A Chartbook* (Menlo Park, CA: Kaiser Family Foundation, 2000), fig 4.7.

34. National Institutes of Health, *FY 2001 Investments,* 2001, www.nih.gov/news/BudgetFY2002/FY2001investments.htm, accessed August 3, 2003.

35. Frank R. Lichtenberg, "Are the Benefits of Newer Drugs Worth Their Cost? Evidence from the 1996 MEPS," *Health Affairs* 20, no. 5 (2001): 241–51.

36. Public Citizen, *The Other Drug War: Big Pharma's 625 Washington Lobbyists,* 2001, www.citizen.org/documents/otherdrugwar.pdf, accessed May 14, 2003; Public Citizen, *Rx Industry Goes for KO: Drug Companies Spend Record Amount This Election Cycle,* 2000, www.citizen.org/congress/reform/drug_industry/contribution/articles.cfm?ID=799, accessed May 14, 2003.

37. Alison Evans Cuellar and Joshua M. Wiener, "Can Social Insurance for Long-Term Care Work? The Experience of Germany," *Health Affairs* 19, no. 3 (2000): 8–25.

38. Laura Summer and Robert Friedland, *The Role of the Asset Test in Targeting Benefits for Medicare Savings Programs* (New York: Commonwealth Fund, 2002).

39. Michael J. Graetz and Jerry L. Mashaw, *True Security: Rethinking American Social Insurance* (New Haven, CT: Yale University Press, 1999).

40. Katherine E. Laws, Roy M. Gabriel, and Bentson H. McFarland, "Integration and Its Discontents: Substance Abuse Treatment in the Oregon Health Plan," *Health Affairs* 21, no. 4 (2002): 284–89.

41. Robert Pear, "Health Providers and Elderly Clash on Medicare Funds: All-Out Lobbying Effort," *New York Times,* May 15, 2000.

42. As described by Representative Sander Levin, Democrat from Michigan, on November 20, 1991, 102nd Cong., 1st sess., *Congressional Record,* http://thomas.loc.gov/home/r102query.html, accessed April 5, 2005.

43. Ibid.

44. Laurel J. Luckholm, Patrick J. Coyne, and Thomas J. Smith, "Palliative Care Program, Medical College of Virginia Campus of Virginia Commonwealth University," in *Pioneer Programs in Palliative Care: Nine Case Studies* (Princeton, NJ: Robert Wood Johnson Foundation and Milbank Memorial Fund, 2000), www.milbank.org/pppc/0011pppc.html#virginia, accessed July 23, 2000.

45. Institute of Medicine, *Extending Medicare Coverage for Preventive and Other Services* (Washington, DC: National Academies Press, 2000).

46. Bureau of National Affairs, *Medicare Report* 11, no. 43 (November 3, 2000).

47. Lynn Wagner, "Novello Bucks White House on Transplant Drugs," *Modern Healthcare,* February 17, 1992.

48. United States Renal Data System, *Annual Data Report/Atlas* (Minneapolis, MN: United States Renal Data System, 2002), table K4.

Chapter 10. Politics

1. Marilyn Moon, *Medicare Now and in the Future,* 2nd ed. (Washington, DC: Urban Institute, 1996), 166.

2. Patricia Neuman and Katheryn M. Langwell, "Medicare's Choice Explosion? Implications for Beneficiaries," *Health Affairs* 18, no. 1 (1999): 150–60.

3. One in ten people over sixty-five and nearly half of those over eighty-five have Alzheimer's. Others have cognitive impairments other than Alzheimer's. See the website of the American Alzheimer's Association, www.alz.org.

4. Jonathan Oberlander, *The Political Life of Medicare* (Chicago: University of Chicago Press, 2003).

5. Theodore Marmor, *The Politics of Medicare,* 2nd ed. (New York: Aldine de Gruyter, 2000), 18.

6. Ibid.

7. Peter Corning, 1969, *The Evolution of Medicare: From Idea to Law,* www.ssa.gov/history/corning.html, accessed June 3, 2003.

8. Eugene Feingold, *Medicare: Policy and Politics* (San Francisco: Chandler, 1966), 59.

9. Quoted in Lawrence R. Jacobs, *The Health of Nations: Public Opinion and the Making of American and British Health Policy* (Ithaca, NY: Cornell University Press, 1993), 150.

10. Edward D. Berkowitz, *Mr. Social Security: The Life of Wilbur J. Cohen* (Lawrence, KS: University Press of Kansas, 1995).

11. Paul Starr, *The Social Transformation of American Medicine* (New York: Basic Books, 1982), 375f.

12. Jacobs, *The Health of Nations,* 149.

13. Associated Press, "Access to Breast Screenings Is Shrinking, Experts Warn," *New York Times,* November 30, 2000.

14. Robert H. Binstock, "A New Era in the Politics of Aging: How Will the Old-Age Interest Groups Respond?" *Generations* 19, no. 3 (1995): 68–74.

15. Feingold, *Medicare: Policy and Politics.*

16. Moon, *Medicare Now and in the Future.*

17. AARP, *NRTA Mission and Vision,* www.aarp.org/nrta, accessed April 5, 2005.

18. Charles R. Morris, *The AARP: America's Most Powerful Lobby and the Clash of Generations* (New York: Times Books, 1996).

19. Ibid.

20. Matthew C. Price, *Justice between Generations: The Growing Power of the Elderly in America* (Westport, CT: Praeger, 1997), 67.

21. Henry J. Pratt, *The Gray Lobby* (Chicago: University of Chicago Press, 1976).

22. Horace Deets, "Building a Strong Tomorrow," *AARP Annual Report,* (Washington, DC: AARP, 1998).

23. Pratt, *The Gray Lobby.*

24. Ibid.

25. Binstock, "A New Era in the Politics of Aging."

26. Pratt, *The Gray Lobby.*

27. Ibid.

28. Kaiser Family Foundation and Harvard School of Public Health, *National Survey on Medicare* (Menlo Park, CA: Kaiser Family Foundation, 1998).

29. Morris, *The AARP*.

30. Christine L. Day, "Old-Age Interest Groups in the 1990s," in *New Directions in Old Age Policies*, ed. Janie S. Steckenrider and Tonya M. Parrott (Albany, NY: State University of New York Press, 1998).

31. Morris, *The AARP*.

32. Ibid.

33. Ibid.

34. Harry Kreisler, 1997, "Conversation with Alan K. Simpson," Institute of International Studies, UC Berkeley, http://Globetrotter.berkeley.edu/conversations/Simpson/simpson6.html, accessed June 2, 2003.

35. James L. Martin, "AARP: Association against Retired Persons," www.members.aol.com/poesgirl/aarp.htm, accessed April 5, 2005.

36. CNN, "Seniors Emerge as Growing Political Force," www.cnn.com/us/9906/29/medicare.recipient, June 29, 1999, accessed April 5, 2005.

37. Binstock, "A New Era in the Politics of Aging."

38. Robert Binstock, Fernando Torres-Gil, and Christine Day have all written on this topic.

39. Christine L. Day, *What Older Americans Think: Interest Groups and Aging Policy* (Princeton, NJ: Princeton University Press, 1990).

40. The Gallup Organization, *Gallup Social and Economic Indicators: The Public and Congress,* 1998, www.gallup.com/poll, accessed April 8, 1999.

41. Network Democracy, *Americans Discuss Social Security,* www.networkdemocracy.org/social-security/bb/whc/adss.html, accessed June 2, 2003.

42. Robert R. Putnam, *Bowling Alone: The Collapse and Revival of American Community* (New York: Simon and Schuster, 2000).

43. Beth Demel and Joseph R. Baker III, "Effects of the Home Health Care Interim Payment System on Access to Home Health Care for People on Medicare," *Care Management Journals* 2, no. 2 (2000): 108–15.

44. Congressional Budget Office, *Budgetary Implications of the Balanced Budget Act of 1997,* December 1997, ftp://ftp.cbo.gov/3xx/doc302/bba-97.pdf, downloaded August 18, 2003.

45. Mary Suther, chairman and chief executive officer, VNA of Texas, Inc., *Testimony before the Finance Committee, United States Senate,* on behalf of the National Association for Home Care, June 10, 1999, www.senate.gov/~finance/6–10 suth.htm, accessed August 19, 2003.

46. National Association for Home Care, *Crisis in Home Care: Dismantling of the Medicare Home Health Benefit,* 2000, www.nahc.org/nahc/legreg/Crisis/crisishh .html, accessed August 18, 2003; U.S. General Accounting Office, *Medicare Home Health Care: Prospective Payment System Could Reverse Recent Declines in Spending,* GAO/HEHS-00–176 (Washington, DC: General Accounting Office, 2000).

47. MedPAC, *Report to the Congress: Medicare Payment Policy* (Washington, DC: MedPAC, 2000).

48. More information about MedPAC can be found at www.medpac.gov.

Chapter 11. Rationing Is Inevitable

1. Lawrence R. Jacobs, *The Health of Nations: Public Opinion and the Making of American and British Health Policy* (Ithaca, NY: Cornell University Press, 1993), 100.

2. The Commonwealth Fund, *Multinational Comparisons of Health Systems Data* (New York: Commonwealth Fund, 2002).

3. Robert Pear, "Health Costs Underestimated: Experts Say Medicare Outlook Dims as Medical Technology Pushes Up Prices," *New York Times,* November 30, 2000; National Academy of Social Insurance, *Financing Medicare's Future* (Washington, DC: National Academy of Social Insurance, 2000); Mark McClellan, *Medicare and the Federal Budget: Past Experience, Current Policy, Future Prospects* (Cambridge, MA: National Bureau of Economic Research, 2000).

4. Rosemary A. Stevens, "Health Care in the Early 1960s," *Health Care Financing Review,* 18 no. 2 (1996): 11–22.

5. MedPAC, *Report to the Congress: Medical Savings Accounts and the Medicare Program* (Washington, DC: Medicare Payment Advisory Commission, 2000).

6. Robert Zussman, *Intensive Care: Medical Ethics and the Medical Profession* (Chicago: University of Chicago Press, 1992).

7. Ian Dey and Neil Fraser, "Age-Based Rationing in the Allocation of Health Care," *Journal of Aging and Health* 12, no. 4 (2000): 511–37.

8. Kaiser Family Foundation, *National Survey of Physicians, Part I: Doctors on Disparities in Medical Care, Highlights and Chartpack* (Menlo Park, CA: Kaiser Family Foundation, 2002).

9. Rudolf Klein, Patricia Day, and Sharon Redmayne, *Managing Scarcity: Priority Setting and Rationing in the NHS* (Buckingham, UK: Open University Press, 1996).

10. Donald M. Berwick, *Escape Fire: Lessons for the Future of Health Care* (New York: Commonwealth Fund, 2002).

11. Mike Clarke, "The Cochrane Collaboration: Providing and Obtaining the Best Evidence about the Effects of Health Care," *Evaluation and the Health Professions* 25, no. 1 (2002): 8–11.

12. Mark H. Eckman, "Patient-Centered Decision Making: A View of the Past and a Look toward the Future," *Medical Decision Making* 21, no. 3 (2001): 241–47.

13. Victor Fuchs and Alan M. Garber, "Medical Innovation: Promises and Pitfalls," *Brookings Review* 21, no. 1 (2003): 44–48.

14. Karen Bloor and Alan Maynard, "Disease Management: A Global Cost-Containing Initiative?" *PharmacoEconomics* 17, no. 6 (2000): 539–44.

15. D. C. Hadorn, "Setting Priorities for Waiting Lists: Defining Our Terms," *Canadian Medical Association Journal* 163, no. 7 (2001): 857–60.

16. D. H. Howard, "Dynamic Analysis of Liver Allocation Policies," *Medical Decision Making* 21, no. 4 (2001): 257–66.

17. J. R. Maurer et al., "International Guidelines for the Selection of Lung Transplant Candidates," *Heart and Lung* 27, no. 4 (1998): 223–29.

18. Institute of Medicine, *Unequal Treatment: Confronting Racial and Ethnic Disparities in Health Care* (Washington, DC: National Academies Press, 2002).

19. Richard D. Lamm and Heather E. Lamm, *The Challenge of an Aging Society* (Denver, CO: Center for Public Policy and Contemporary Issues, University of Denver, 1996); Daniel Callahan, "Limiting Health Care for the Old," in *Aging and Ethics*, ed. Nancy S. Jecker (Clifton, NJ: Humana Press, 1991).

20. Zussman, *Intensive Care.*

21. Dey and Fraser, "Age-Based Rationing."

Chapter 12. The Social Contract

1. Social Security Administration, *A Brief History of Social Security,* www.ssa.gov/history/briefhistory3.html, accessed June 10, 2003.

2. Abraham Epstein, *Insecurity: A Challenge to America,* 3rd ed. (New York: Random House, 1936).

3. Daniel Fox, personal correspondence, October 20, 2000.

4. Walter I. Trattner, *From Poor Law to Welfare State: A History of Social Welfare in America,* 6th ed. (New York: Free Press, 1999).

5. Social Security Administration, *Social Security History,* www.ssa.gov/history/history6.html, accessed March 31, 2003.

6. Quoted by E. J. Dionne, "Social Insurance Commentary," in *Medicare: Preparing for the Challenges of the 21st Century,* ed. Robert D. Reischauer, Stuart Butler, and Judith Lave (Washington, DC: Brookings Institution Press, 1998), 39.

7. See, for example, E. Kimbark MacColl, with Harry M. Stern, *Merchants, Money, and Power: The Portland Establishment, 1843–1913* (Portland, OR: Georgian Press, 1988).

8. James Weinstein, *The Corporate Ideal in the Liberal State, 1900–1918* (Boston: Beacon, 1968).

9. David Caute, *The Great Fear: The Anti-Communist Purge under Truman and Eisenhower* (New York: Simon and Schuster, 1978).

10. Elizabeth Warren, Teresa Sullivan, and Melissa Jacoby, "Medical Problems and Bankruptcy Filings," *Norton's Bankruptcy Adviser,* May 2000, http://papers.ssrn.com/sol3/papers.cfm?abstract_id=224581, accessed June 9, 2003; Teresa A. Sullivan, Elizabeth Warren, and Jay L. Westbrook, *The Fragile Middle Class: Americans in Debt* (New Haven, CT: Yale University Press, 2000); David U. Himmelstein, Elizabeth Warren, Deborah Thorne, and Steffie Woolhandler, "Market Watch: Illness and Injury as Contributors to Bankruptcy," *Health Affairs* Web Exclusive, February 2, 2005, www.healthaffairs.org/WebExclusives.php, accessed April 4, 2005.

11. Robert J. Blendon et al., "Common Concerns amid Diverse Systems: Health Care Experiences in Five Countries," *Health Affairs* 22, no. 3 (2003): 106–21; Kaiser Family Foundation, *Kaiser HealthPoll Report: Health Security Watch,* March–April 2003, www.kff.org/healthpollreport, accessed June 9, 2003.

12. National Public Radio, Kaiser Family Foundation, and Kennedy School of Government, *Toplines: National Survey of Americans' Views on Taxes,* 2003, www.kff.org and www.npr.org, accessed June 9, 2003.

13. Carsten G. Ullrich, "Reciprocity, Justice and Statutory Health Insurance in Germany," *Journal of European Social Policy* 12, no. 2 (2002): 123–36.

14. Daniel Kahneman, Jack L. Knetsch, and Richard Thaler, "Fairness as a Constraint on Profit Seeking, Entitlements in the Market," *American Economic Review* 76, no. 4 (1986): 728–41.

15. Colin F. Camerer, *Behavioral Game Theory: Experiments in Strategic Interaction* (New York: Russell Sage Foundation, 2003).

16. NPR, Kaiser Family Foundation, and Kennedy School, *Toplines.*

17. Jack Hadley and John Holahan, "How Much Medical Care Do the Uninsured Use, and Who Pays for It?" *Health Affairs* web exclusive, February 12, 2003, http://content.healthaffairs.org/cgi/content/full/hlthaff.w3.66vi/DC1, accessed March 15, 2005.

18. President's Commission for the Study of Ethical Problems in Medicine and Biomedical and Behavioral Research, *Securing Access to Health Care: A Report on the Ethical Implications of Differences in the Availability of Health Services* (Washington, DC: Government Printing Office, 1983).

19. Karien Stronks et al., "Who Should Decide? Qualitative Analysis of Panel Data from Public, Patients, Healthcare Professionals, and Insurers on Priorities in Health Care," *British Medical Journal* 315 (July 12, 1997): 92–96.

20. Edward L. Lascher, Jr. and Michael R. Powers, eds., *The Economics and Politics of No-Fault Insurance* (Boston: Kluwer, 2001); Jeffrey O'Connell, *Ending Insult to Injury: No-Fault Insurance for Products and Services* (Chicago: University of Illinois Press, 1975).

21. Michael J. Graetz and Jerry L. Mashaw, *True Security* (New Haven, CT: Yale University Press, 1999).

22. P. Wynand et al., "Risk Adjustment and Risk Selection on the Sickness Fund Insurance Market in Five European Countries," *Health Policy* (2002): 1–24.

23. David M. Cutler and Ellen Meara, "The Concentration of Medical Spending: An Update," working paper 7279 (Cambridge, MA: National Bureau of Economic Research, 1999).

24. James Lubitz et al., "Three Decades of Health Care Use by the Elderly, 1965–1998," *Health Affairs* 20, no. 2 (2001): 19–32; Norman G. Levinsky et al., "Influence of Age on Medicare Expenditures and Medical Care in the Last Year of Life," *Journal of the American Medical Association* 286, no. 11 (2001): 1349–55; Donald R. Hoover et al., "Medical Expenditures during the Last Year of Life: Findings from the 1992–1996 Medicare Current Beneficiary Survey," *Health Services Research* 37, no. 6 (2002):1625–42.

25. Kaiser Family Foundation, *Medicare Chartbook* (Menlo Park, CA: Kaiser Family Foundation, 2001); Allen R. Nissenson and Richard A. Rettig, "Medicare's End-Stage Renal Disease Program: Current Status and Future Prospects," *Health Affairs* 18, no. 1 (1999): 161–79.

26. Jagadeesh Gokhale and Laurence J. Kotlikoff, "Medicare from the Per-

spective of Generational Accounting," in Andrew Rettenmaier and Thomas Saving, eds., *Medicare Reform: Issues and Answers* (Chicago: University of Chicago Press, 1999), 153–73. The countries compared were France, Germany, Italy, Canada, Japan, and the United States.

27. Robert M. Ball, "Perspectives on Medicare: What Medicare's Architects Had in Mind," *Health Affairs* 14, no. 4 (1995): 62–72.

Index

Indexer:	Patricia Deminna
Compositor:	Binghamton Valley Composition, LLC
Text:	10/13 Galliard
Display:	Galliard
Printer and binder:	Maple-Vail Manufacturing Group